THE BIG BOOK OF

Braiding

55 ELEGANT AND STYLISH BRAIDS FOR EVERY OCCASION

BY PETER HÄGELSTAM AND HELÉN PELLBÄCK

WITH ALINA BALOGH, SALIOU BARRY, AND SOFIA GEIDEBY

PHOTOGRAPHS BY LEONARD GREN AND MARCUS FRIXSON

TEXT BY DANIELLE DEASISMONT

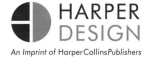

HARPER DESIGN

An Imprint of HarperCollinsPublishers

Originally published in 2015 in Sweden as *Den stora boken om flätor.*

THE BIG BOOK OF BRAIDING.
Copyright © 2015 by Bokförlaget Max Ström.
English translation © 2016 by HarperCollins Publishers.

HarperCollins books may be purchased for educational, business, or sales promotional use. For information please e-mail the Special Markets Department at SPsales@harpercollins.com.

First published in 2016 by
Harper Design,
An Imprint of HarperCollins*Publishers*
195 Broadway
New York, NY 10007
Tel: (212) 207-7000
Fax: 855-746-6023
harperdesign@harpercollins.com
www.hc.com

This edition distributed throughout the world by:
HarperCollinsPublishers
195 Broadway
New York, NY 10007

Library of Congress Control Number: 2016940708

ISBN 978-0-06-249907-3

First Printing, 2016

Printed and bound by Livonia in Latvia

Text: Danielle Deasismont
Cover photo and inspirational images: Leonard Gren
Instructional photographs: Marcus Erixson
Typography and design: Patric Leo
Original and layout: Anna Hild
Illustrations: Peter Hägelstam
Hairstylists: Peter Hägelstam, Helén Pellbäck, Alina Balogh, Saliou Barry, and Sofia Geideby
Project leader and stylist: Helén Pellbäck
Makeup: Jenny Karlsson
Reprography: JK Morris, Värnamo

Contents

Introduction

Many of us have special memories associated with braids. Maybe someone braided your hair for the first day of school, or maybe you used to braid your dolls' hair when you were little. Throughout time and across cultures, families and friends have gathered together around braiding as a way to socialize. Braiding is not only a way to create beautiful hairstyles but also brings people together and makes them engage with each other. When you braid someone's hair, it can lead to conversation and connection, a way to get to know each other a little better.

People have always used hair as an important way to express identity, and the craft of braiding is one of the oldest in the world. Some scholars believe that the 20,000-year-old limestone figurine known as Venus of Willendorf, an icon of prehistoric art, is wearing a braided hairstyle, and the striking braids that we call cornrows today can be found in 5,000-year-old images from the Sahara. The history of the braid is thus a long one.

Hairstyles can also be expressions of religious and political climate. A present-day example is that of the former Ukrainian prime minister, Yulia Tymoshenko, whose famous braid became an important part of her public image. Our hair's appearance says a great deal about us and about the times in which we live.

The braid has an important function in creating a variety of hairstyles and is not only beautiful but also practical. Braiding is a good tool for putting hair up in a bun, keeping long strands together, or dealing with wisps that can get in the way. Braids can serve as the foundation for a more elaborate hairstyle, and hair ornaments or flowers can also easily be fastened to a braid when creating an updo. Braided hairstyles spark interest. They can look intricate yet still have a simple design that is easy to create. The contemporary braid expresses and enhances your style for the day; you can begin with a sleek, smooth, and classic braid, and then pull it apart for a more bohemian look.

Over the years, braiding has always been a part of fashion trends, in one way or another. From the voluminous braid of the 1960s to the swinging hippie braids of the 1970s, braiding styles have followed the trendy hair lengths. In folklore and art as well, braids have played an important role. Pippi Longstocking, Rapunzel, and now Elsa from Disney's *Frozen* have all given a face to the braid. The iconic Scandinavian fairies, elves, and forest trolls found in the paintings of Swedish artist John Bauer are often portrayed with long flowing hair and braids; and the Mexican painter Frida Kahlo usually depicted herself with braids in her famous self-portraits, making them part of her signature look.

Many style icons and celebrities have inspired us with their hairstyles. The actresses Elizabeth Taylor and Grace Kelly wore many elegant braided styles created by the legendary stylist Alexandre de Paris. Today as well, braided coiffures are often seen on the red carpet. Rihanna, Nicole Kidman, Blake Lively, and Paris Hilton are among the many celebrities who have appeared recently with braided styles.

In this book, we share some of our favorite hairstyles. Some are stylish classics, while others have a more advanced, avant-garde-inspired form. Sometimes the braid can make up the entire hairstyle, or it can be just one detail. Half a head of braided hair, or braids on one side, for example, can become striking details in your look. The best thing about braids is that even the simplest varieties can make a strong impact. You can make infinite variations with braids, the only limit being your imagination. Here you will find styles at every level of difficulty and presented on different types and lengths of hair.

No two braids are alike, and you can always find new ways to transform the braid so that it fits your own personal style. Try pulling your braid apart, pulling loosely for a more feathery look, or hard enough to loosen individual strands. You can divide the hair into multiple small sections with parts that curve, and create patterns on the head, or you can alternate tight and loose rounds in order to design your own braided style.

We hope you'll be inspired when you open this book. Dare to experiment with new braiding techniques and make every hairstyle your own.

Good luck!
Peter Hägelstam and Helén Pellbäck at Björn Axén Academy

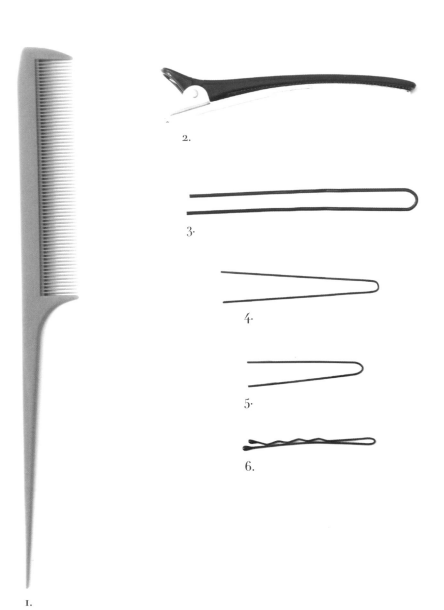
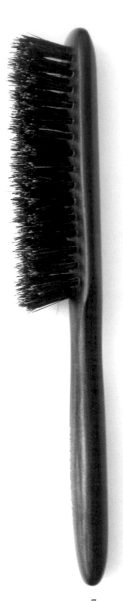

1.

2.

3.

4.

5.

6.

7.

Tools

1. Rattail comb

2. Hair clips

3. Sturdy, extra long hairpins

4. Long hairpins

5. Short hairpins

6. Bobby pins

7. Hairbrush, preferably with boar bristles

   Saltwater spray

   Hairspray, one with firm hold and one with light hold

   Elastic bands, different sizes

   Shine cream

Glossary

Anchor point: A place where the braid can be secured using pins. An anchor point can be a ponytail or a strand of hair that has been teased.

Crimp: To treat the hair with a crimper or small waver.

Before you begin braiding

To achieve the best results with your hairstyle, it is important to start out with freshly washed hair before you begin braiding. Hair that has just been washed can sometimes be slippery and hard to style, but by preparing it with the right products it will be easier to work with.

Prepare the hair by dampening it with a saltwater spray. Then dry the hair with a blow-dryer. Any whorls and small waves at the roots of the hair can be straightened by brushing as you blow-dry the hair. Saltwater spray makes the hair a little coarser and fuller, which makes it easier to create the hairstyle. If you want your braids to look fuller, you can also use a crimping iron after applying saltwater spray. If you choose to crimp the hair, make sure not to squeeze the iron too hard since that can leave marks. You can also tease the hair strand before you crimp it, which will give the strand a lighter wave.

Brush through the hair thoroughly before you begin braiding to prevent tangles.

As you braid

Divide the hair into different sections as you braid. This will make it easier to keep track of what needs to be braided and when. Use hair clips to keep the sections separated.

It is a good idea to use hairspray with a lighter hold while you work. Avoid spray products with a pump, as they can make the hair too wet.

To create a fuller hairstyle you can pull at the braid. Take hold of it with your thumb and forefinger and pull carefully at the braid, in an up-and-down direction. Using this technique you can create different styles, a sloppy braid or a tight one. For a tighter and more controlled braid, you can use a shine cream to keep small hairs in place.

Create a style with staying power

In order to make your hairstyle long-lasting, you need to have anchor points that you can use to keep it stable. A good anchor point can be a ponytail, a teased strand of hair, or a hair clip that is fastened into the style.

Use long hairpins while you are experimenting with your style. You can easily remove the pins and reposition the anchor point if you aren't satisfied with it. Don't forget to look at your hairstyle both in profile and from the back. When you are finished and want to fasten your hair sections, you can replace the hairpins with bobby pins.

When you use bobby pins to secure the hair, push the pin into the hair with a circular movement so that you can grab underlying hair to use as an anchor.

When the style is completed, you can finish with a stiffer hairspray to get more stability. It is hard to change the hairstyle after you have used a stiffer spray, so only do this as a final step once you are completely satisfied with the hairstyle.

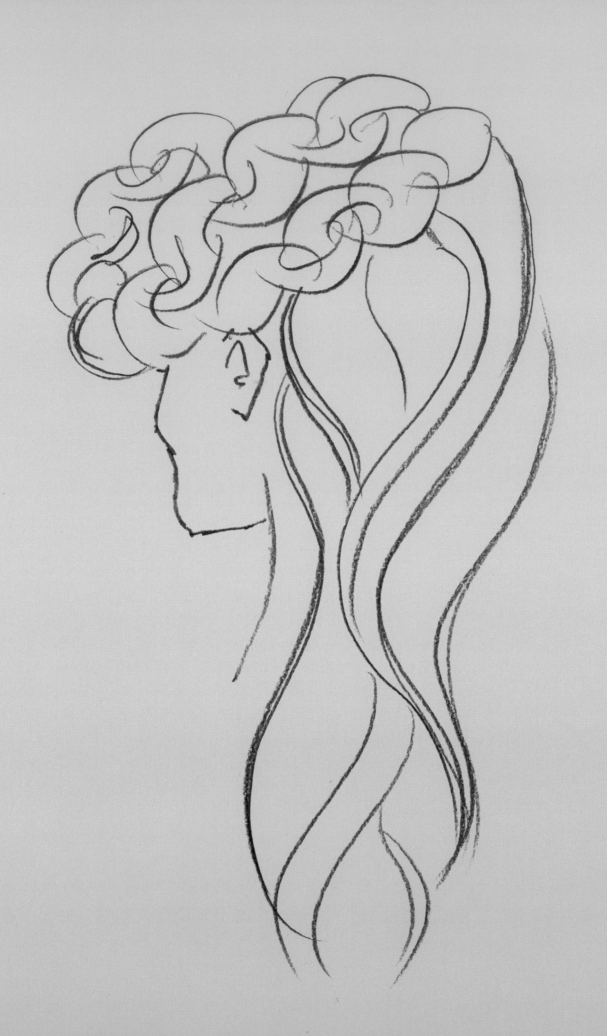

French Braids

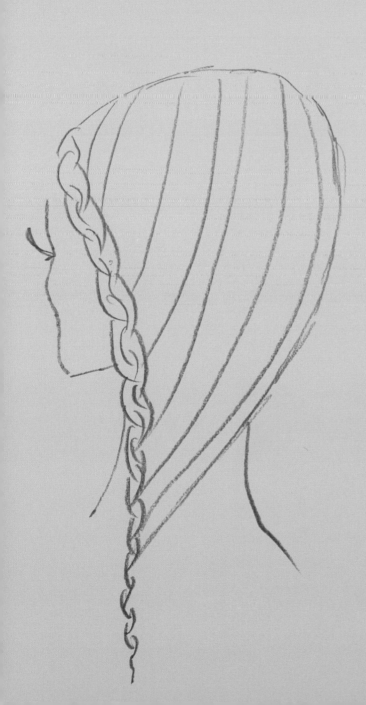

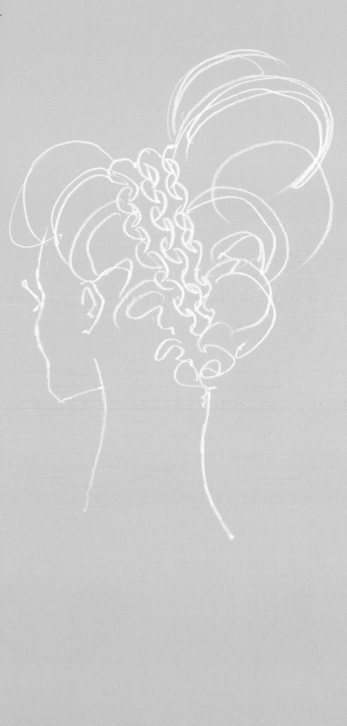

Classic French Braid

A practical braid that breathes romance, the French braid is also a good everyday style because it's so easy to create.

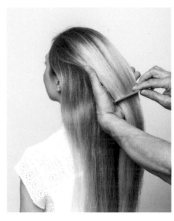

1. Brush the hair, pulling it back toward the neck.

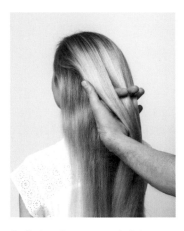

2. Gather the topmost hair into a teardrop-shaped section. Divide the section into three strands using your fingers.

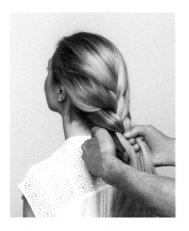

3. Begin making the French braid. First make one round of a basic braid, crossing each side strand over the center strand. After this first round, add in more hair from the side every time you cross a side strand over the center.

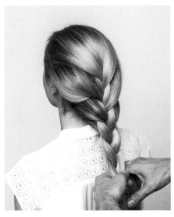

4. Continue to alternate right and left sides, picking up additional strands each time so that you keep adding to each section of hair. Repeat until the entire length of hair is braided.

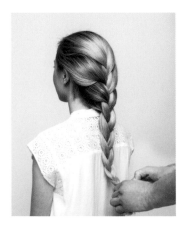

5. Fasten with an elastic.

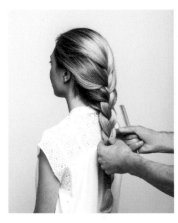

6. Gently pull at the braid to create more volume.

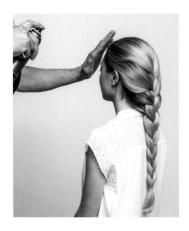

7. Smooth any stray hairs into place using hairspray.

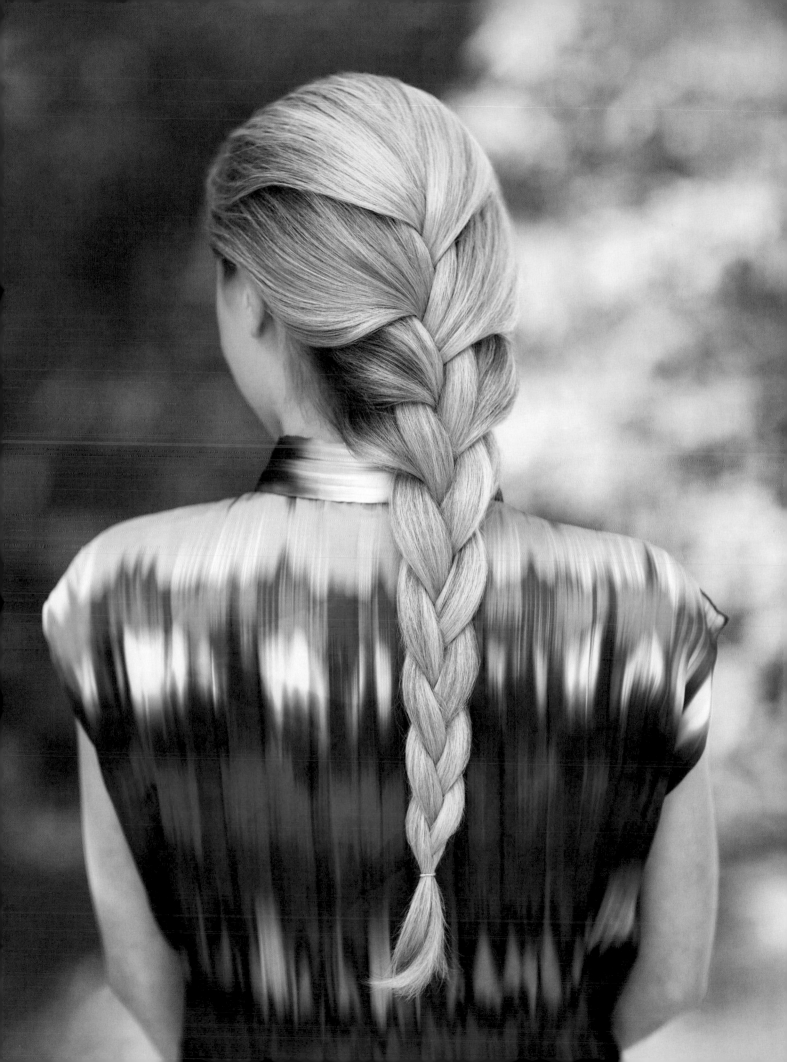

Edge Braid

A simple yet elegant hairstyle, this half French braid gathers the hair on one shoulder. Perfect for every day!

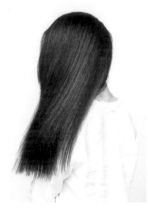

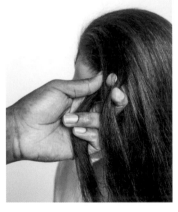

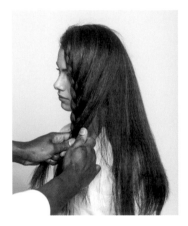

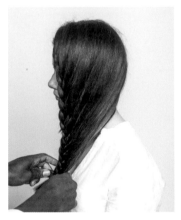

1. Brush the hair to one side. You can use a shine cream to achieve the smoothest, shiniest surface possible. This hairstyle consists of a half French braid that starts from the bangs.

2. Take a small section of hair from the bangs and divide into three strands. Make one round of a basic braid, crossing the side strands over the center strand. Then add in a new section of hair from one outside edge for each new crossover.

3. Continue braiding, but only add in hair from one side. Repeat until the entire length is braided. The braid should go alongside the face. Try to keep your hands down as you braid to get more weight in the braid.

4. Fasten with a thin elastic.

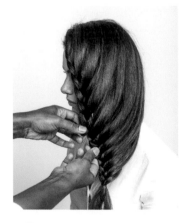

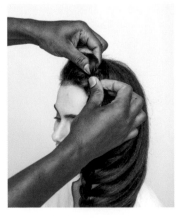

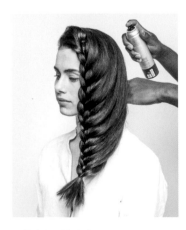

5. For a softer feel, pull at the braid with your fingers.

6. Lift up the braid at the forehead and fasten with a hairpin.

7. Finish with hairspray.

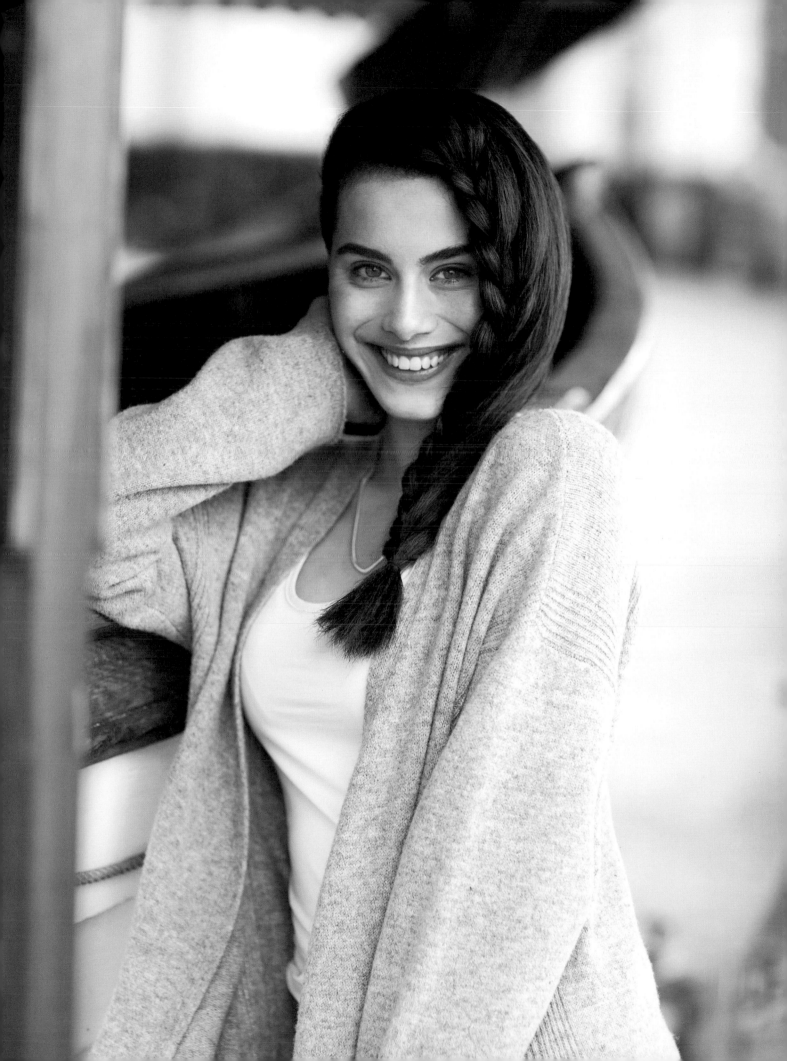

Elsa

The Elsa is a romantic hairstyle with a half French braid that sweeps over one shoulder. Think of braiding loosely and airily in order to add volume to the braid.

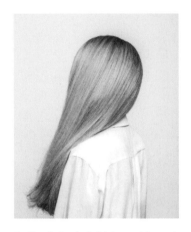

1. Brush the hair. Make a side part. Gather all the hair in front of one shoulder.

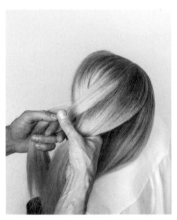

2. Separate a large section of hair at the top of the head and make a half French braid. Divide the hair into three strands. First make one round of a basic braid. Then add in a new strand of hair from one outside edge for each new crossover.

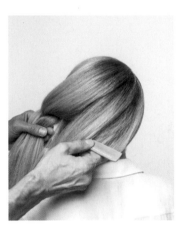

3. Continue braiding, but only add in new hair from one side.

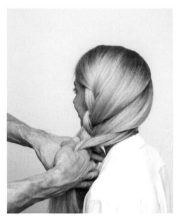

4. Add in large chunks of hair to achieve a thick and full braid. Always braid downward, toward the shoulder. Fasten with an elastic.

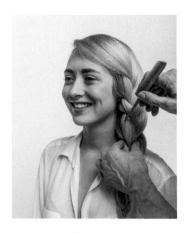

5. Use the tail of a comb to gather in any stray hairs.

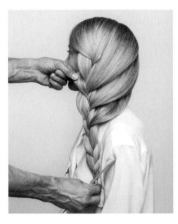

6. Now tug carefully at the braid. Hold the ends while you tug to keep the braid from dissolving.

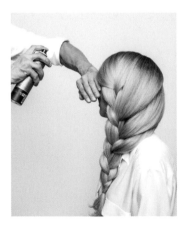

7. Finish with hairspray.

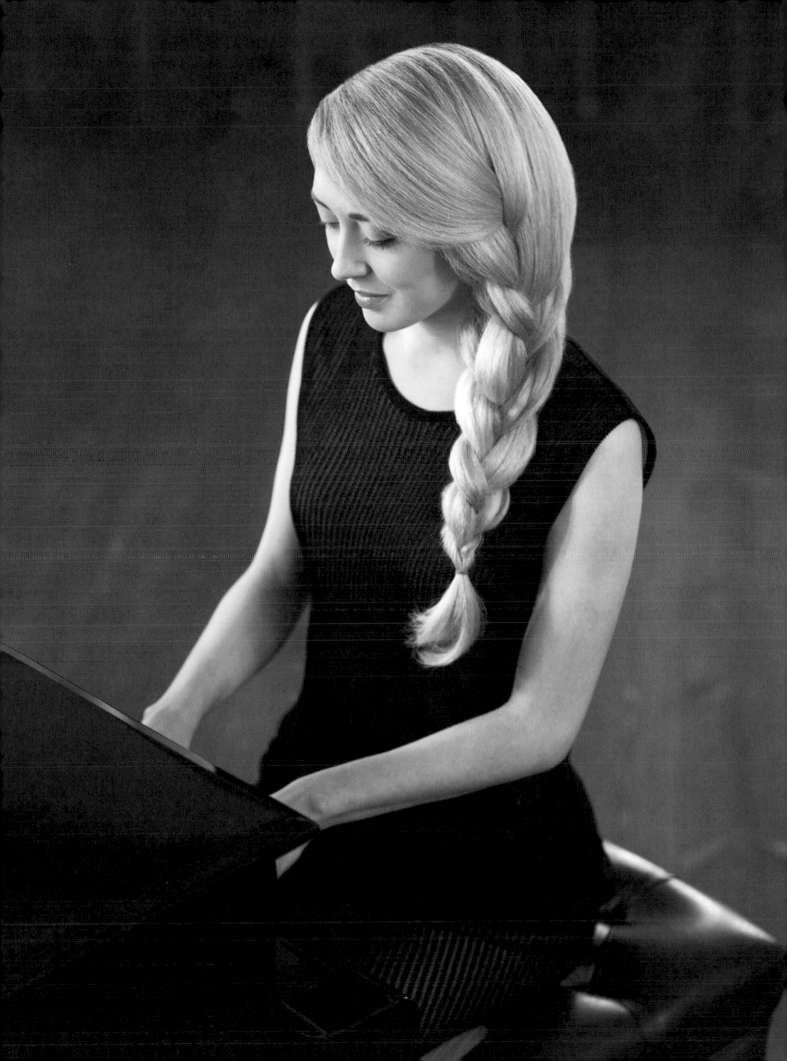

Beret

A style that evokes the 1920s, this updo features two French braids that melt into each other.

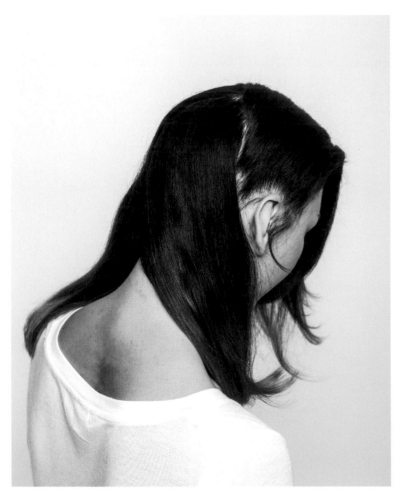

1. Part the hair, beginning just behind the ear and moving up toward the middle of the crown. Brush the front hair section down toward the opposite eye.

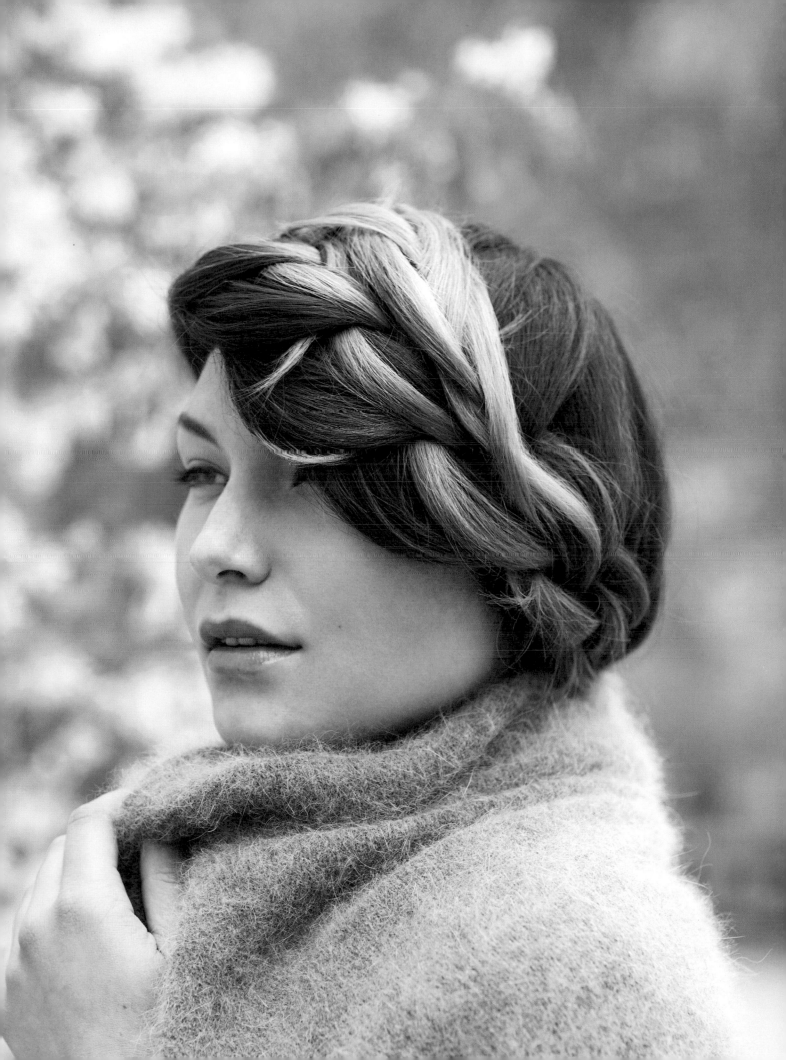

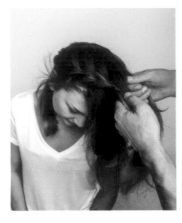

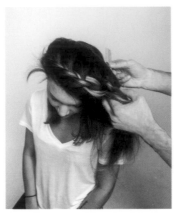

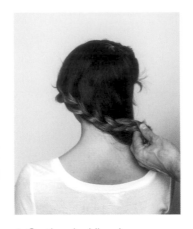

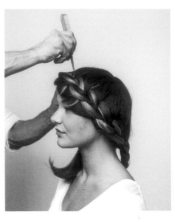

2. Make a French braid. First make one round of a basic braid, where the side strands are crossed over the middle strand. After the first round, pick up a new strand from the outer edge each time you make a new crossover. Braid loosely in order to create a full braid.

3. Alternate right and left sides by picking up new strands of hair and adding to each section.

4. Continue braiding down toward the ear, and then curve the braid across the neck and toward the other side of the face. Braid the entire length. Fasten with an elastic.

5. Pull at the braid until you achieve the desired look.

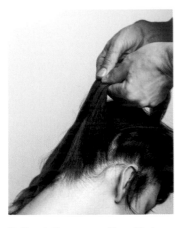

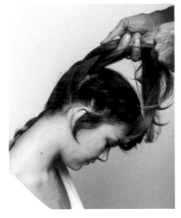

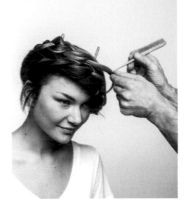

6. Brush the rear section of hair upward.

7. Make a French braid that goes up toward the crown, using the same technique as described in steps 2 and 3.

8. Fasten the braid temporarily with hairpins. Using the tail of a comb, pull out strands of hair from the braid until you achieve the desired feel. Secure the braid with hairpins.

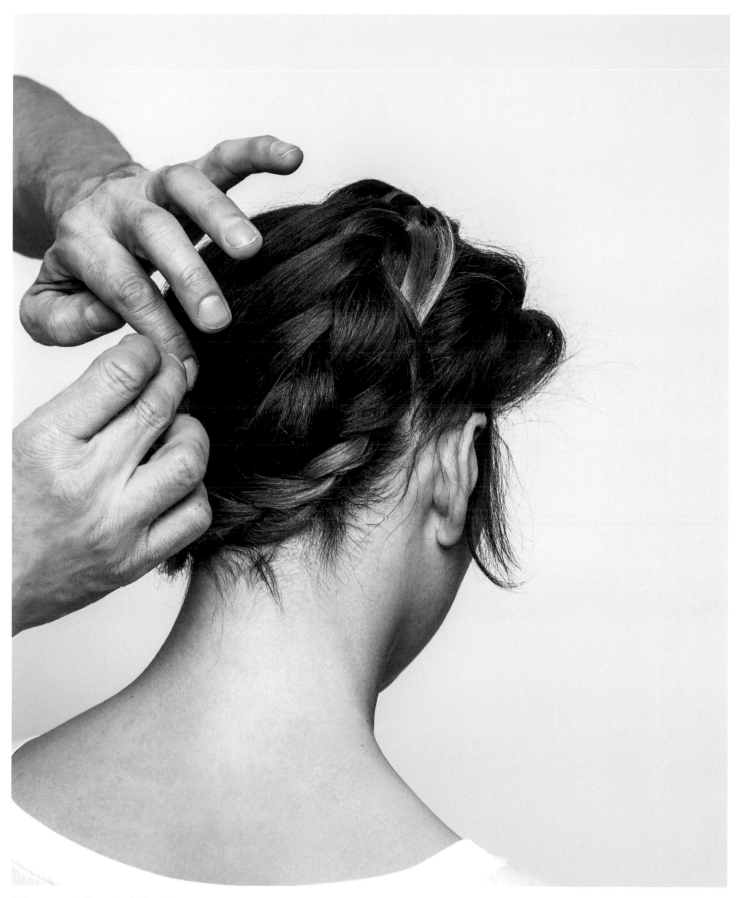

9. Integrate the lower braid into the upper one
using hairpins. Finish with hairspray.

Braided Beret

This style is reminiscent of a knitted beret. Think of braiding airily so that the style has lots of volume.

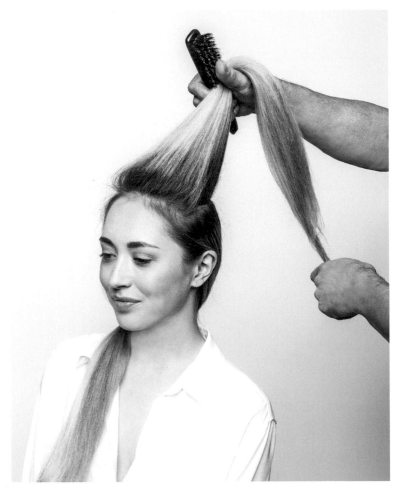

1. Divide the hair into two sections, one at the crown of the head and one below. Gather the lower section of hair into a ponytail and pull it in front of the shoulder.

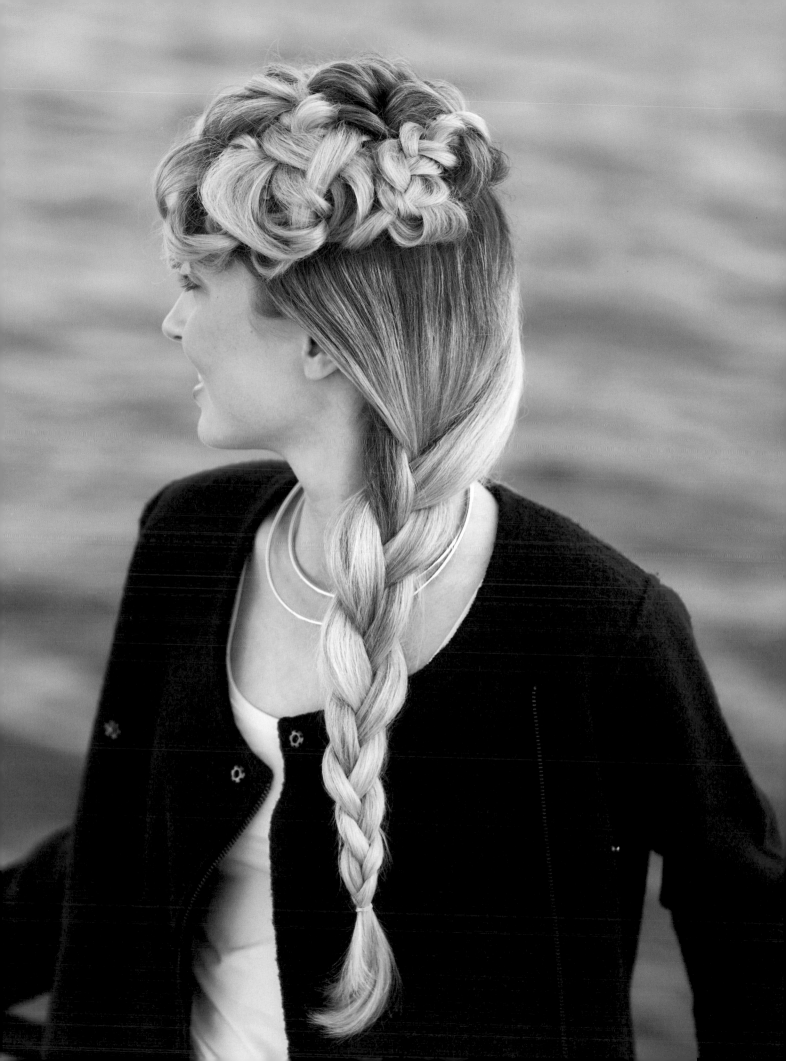

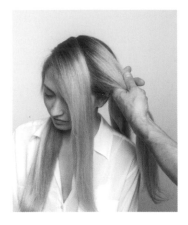

2. Comb the crown hair forward toward the face. Divide it into three large sections.

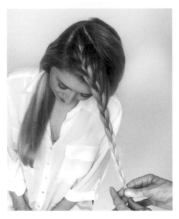

3. Make a French braid from the section nearest the face and divide into three subsections. First make one round of a basic braid, crossing the side strands over the middle strand. Pick up a new section of hair from the outside edges with each new crossover. Alternate right and left sides by picking up new strands and adding to each section. Repeat until the entire length of hair is braided.

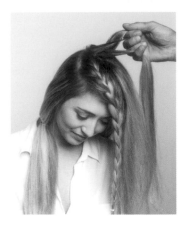

4. Now continue to the center section. Repeat the same braid as in step 3.

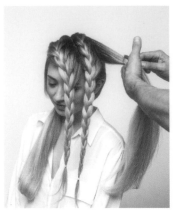

5. Finish with the third section, repeating the same braid as in step 3.

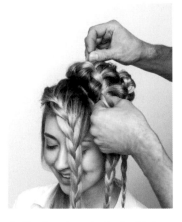

6. Create volume in the braids by using hairpins. Use a hairpin to lift the braid, rotate and fasten at the crown.

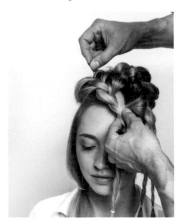

7. Repeat step 6 for all three braids.

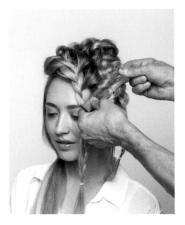

8. Pull at the braids to create a relaxed look. Expand the braids as much as possible.

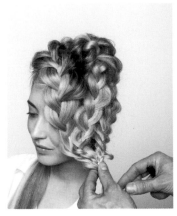

9. Gather all three braids together.

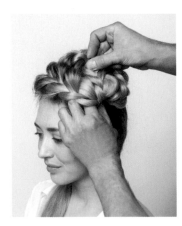

10. Roll the ends in toward the scalp. Use hairpins to fasten the braids, making sure that the elastics are hidden.

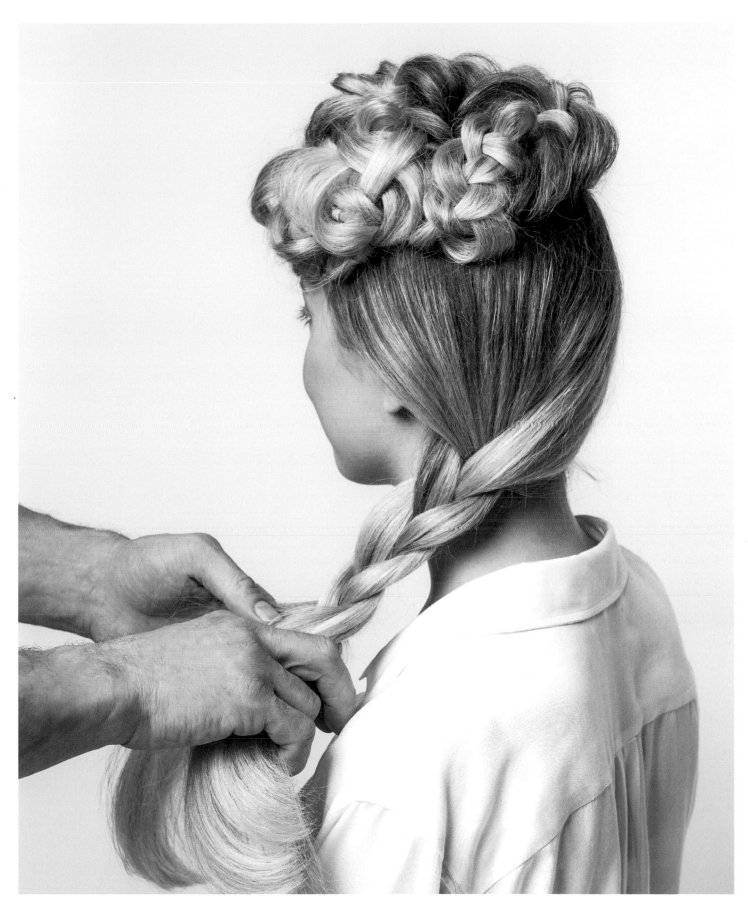

11. Now gather the lower section of hair on the same side as the braids. Divide this section into three smaller sections. Make a regular three-strand braid. Fasten with a thin elastic.

Mohican Braid

This is a French braid with plenty of volume and height that ends in a simple ponytail. Stylish and classic!

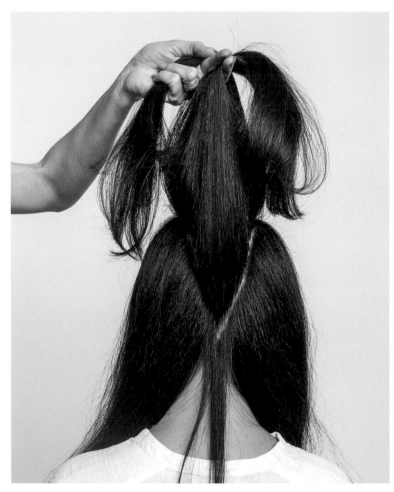

1. Part the hair in the shape of a V from the center of the forehead down toward the back of the head. Also make a V-shaped part from the nape of the neck up toward the back part of the head. Together the two parts will form a diamond shape. Separate out a thin strand at the neck.

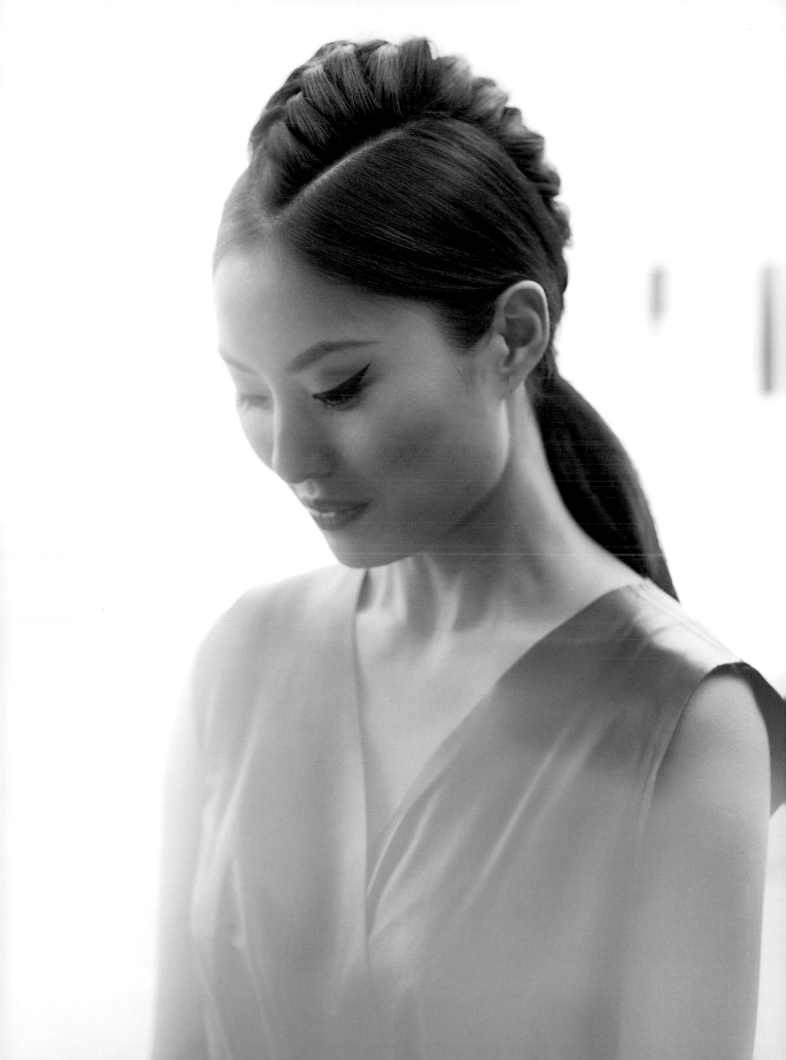

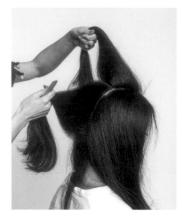

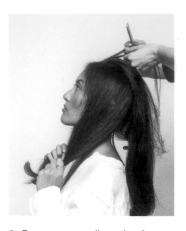

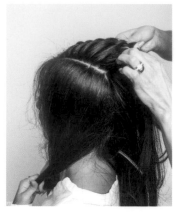

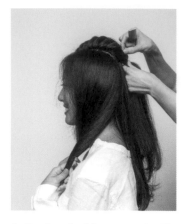

2. Divide the upper and lower sections of hair. Gather the lower section and fasten with a hair clip. Comb the upper hair back toward the neck.

3. Separate a small section from the upper hair at the hairline. Divide this section into three strands, then make one round of a basic braid, where side strands cross over the middle strand. Pick up a new strand with each new crossing.

4. Alternate right and left sides by adding in new strands of hair to each section. Braid upward, away from the scalp, to make the braid airy and porous.

5. Continue braiding upward until you reach the top of the head. Fasten the braid with a small hairpin to secure the height before you continue braiding.

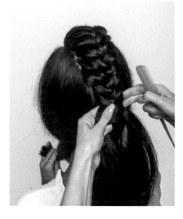

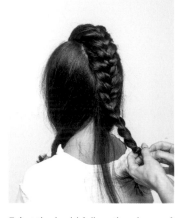

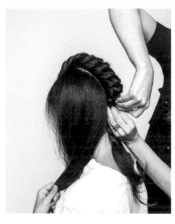

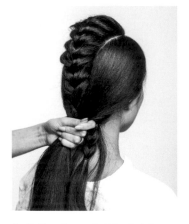

6. Continue braiding with the same technique, airy and porous.

7. Let the braid follow the shape of the head down toward the neck. Fasten with an elastic.

8. Lift up the braid in order to create more height. Secure the height by rotating a hairpin into the braid, and fasten at the neck.

9. Gather the rest of the hair from the sides and brush it smooth against the neck. Gather it into a ponytail as close to the head as possible, using your hands. Leave a small strand at the neck free.

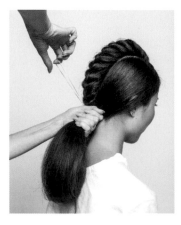

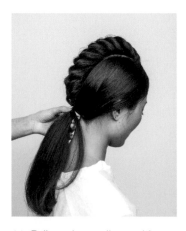

10. Fasten the ponytail with an elastic, winding it tightly for stability.

11. Pull out the small strand from underneath the braid. Wrap the strand around the elastic so that it is covered.

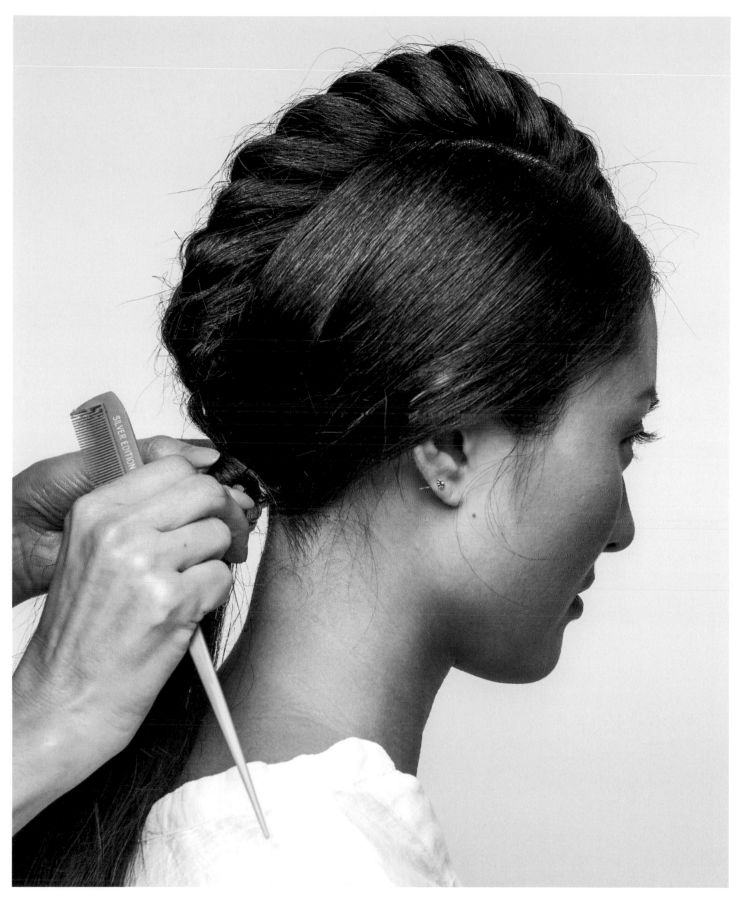

12. Fasten the strand with a hairpin. Finish with hairspray.

Romantic Hat Braid

This style gives the illusion of a big hat resting on your head. The French braid is airy and porous, which lends it a romantic feel.

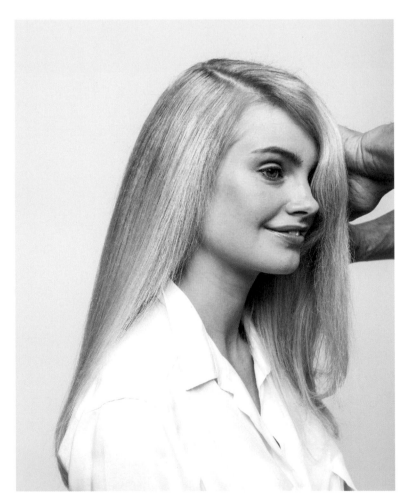

1. Brush through all the hair. Part at the side using a rattail comb.

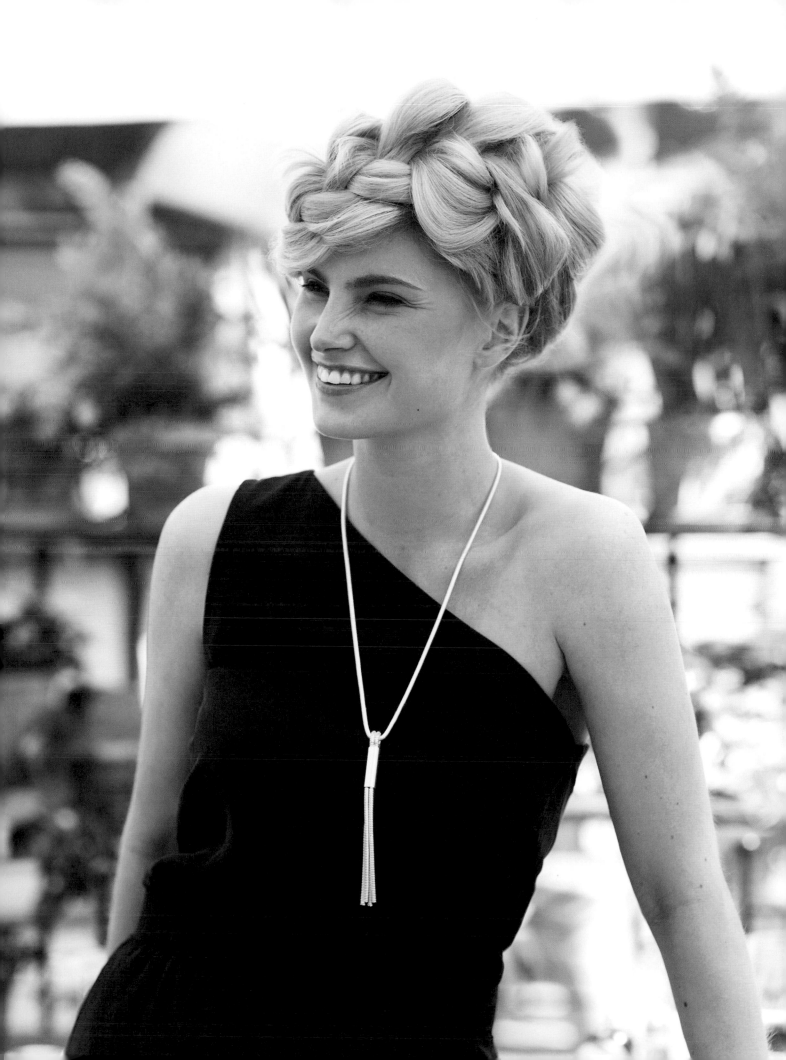

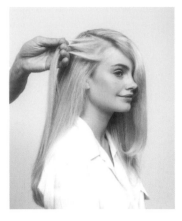

2. Now you will make a French braid that follows the shape of the head. Separate a small section closest to the part and divide into three strands with your fingers.

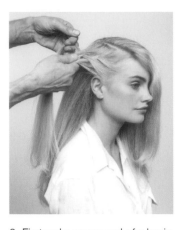

3. First make one round of a basic braid, where the side strands are crossed over the middle strand. After the first round, pick up a new strand from the outside edges each time you make a new crossover.

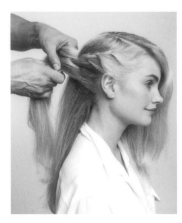

4. Alternate right and left sides by adding in new strands of hair to each section.

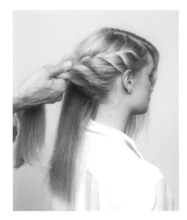

5. Braid with a loose hand, keeping the braid relaxed. The braid will keep growing bigger as you integrate more hair into it.

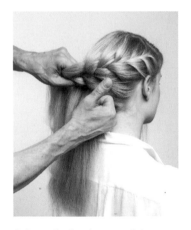

6. It can be hard to get all the hair into the braid. Hair that will not stay in, such as the hair at the neck, can be left to fall naturally for a relaxed feeling. The same goes for any ends that may stick out.

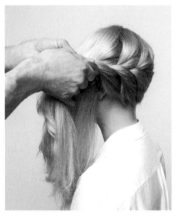

7. Continue braiding the entire length of hair, working your way around the head.

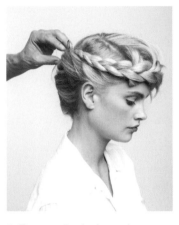

8. Temporarily pin the ends.

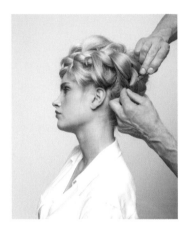

9. Lift up the thickest part of the braid and fasten using extra-long hairpins.

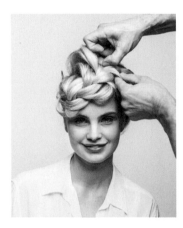

10. Pull at the braid as much as it will tolerate, experimenting until you achieve the look that you want. Let the braid rest over the forehead.

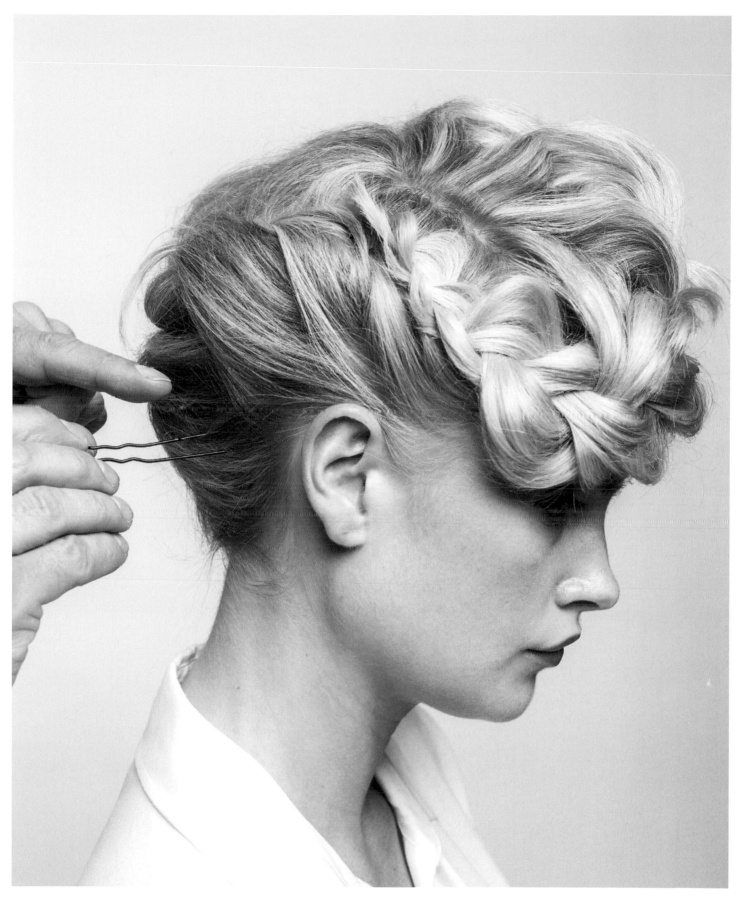

11. Fasten the end of the braid to the root of the braid, using a small hairpin. Finish with hairspray.

Lively Gala Braid

This messy updo combines several different types of braids. In order to get the right feel, we tease the ends, which adds some attitude to the hairstyle.

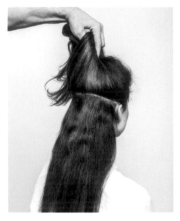

1. Make a part from ear to ear, so that you have two sections. Clip the upper section out of the way. Then divide the lower section of the hair in the middle, making two subsections.

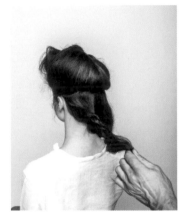

2. Divide the left section into two strands. Twist the right strand inward. Switch sides by twisting the left strand over the right one. Twist the right strand inward. Switch sides again and repeat to create a rope-shaped braid.

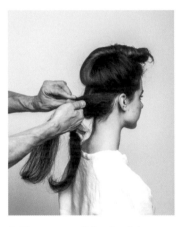

3. Repeat step 2 for the right section.

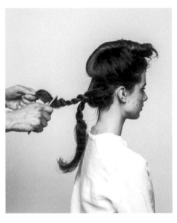

4. Tease the hair hard with a comb in order to secure the braids, and set with hairspray.

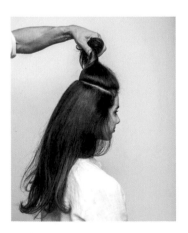

5. Unclip the upper section of hair and draw another part from temple to temple in the shape of a half circle. Clip the crown hair out of the way. Divide the midsection into two parts so that you can start making two French braids.

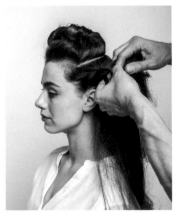

6. The braid should start at the ear and run alongside the head on the left side. First make one round of a basic braid, where the side strands are crossed over the middle strand. After the first round, pick up a new strand from the outside edges each time you make a new crossover.

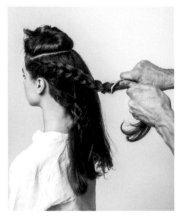

7. Alternate right and left sides of the braid by adding in new strands of hair to each section. Braid the length and then tease hard to secure the braid.

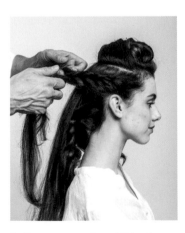

8. Repeat steps 6 and 7 for the right section.

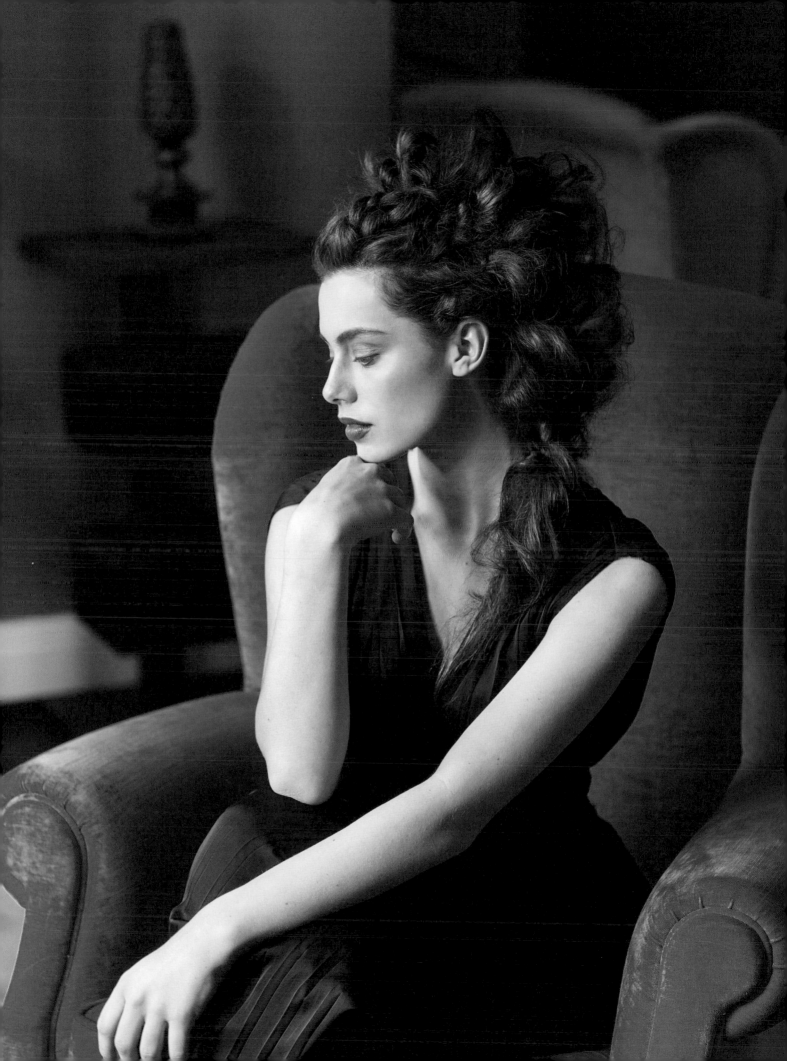

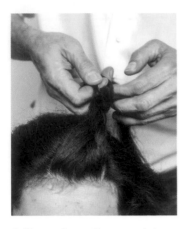

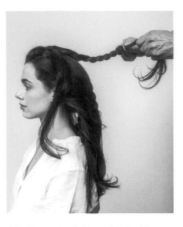

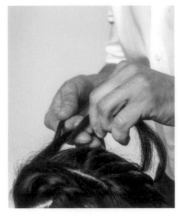

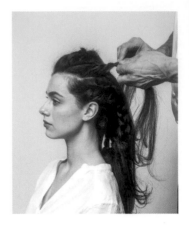

9. Now unfasten the crown hair. Separate a small section at the center of the forehead. Make a French braid by repeating step 6.

10. Alternate right and left sides by picking up new strands of hair and adding to each section. Braid half the length and then tease hard to secure the braid.

11. Make a rope braid using one section in the middle. Begin at the front and divide the hair into two subsections. Always twist the right strand inward. Switch sides by twisting the left strand over the right. Switch sides again and repeat. Leave one-third of the length unbraided.

12. To the left of the French braid, make another French braid with the remaining hair. Braid using the same technique described in steps 9 and 10. Leave a third of the length unbraided. Tease the ends to secure braids.

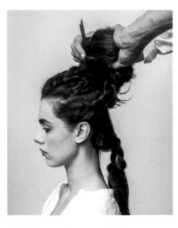

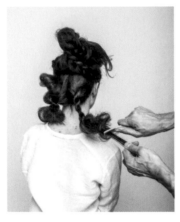

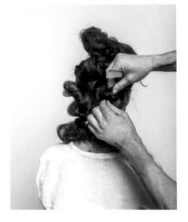

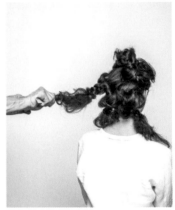

13. Lift up all except the lowest braids. Fasten with a hair clip.

14. Now work with the undermost braids. Tease the ends roughly and pull at the braid to create a dramatic look.

15. Lift the braids onto the head and fasten with hairpins.

16. Unfasten the braids in the middle. Tease the ends roughly and pull at the braids for a dramatic look.

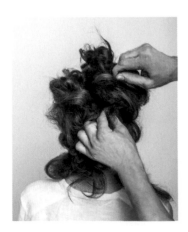

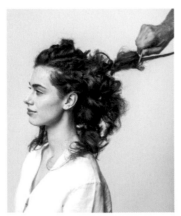

17. Lift the braids and fasten with hairpins.

18. Unfasten the braids at the crown. Tease the ends roughly and pull at the braids to create more texture. Tease the braids at the top of the head more softly.

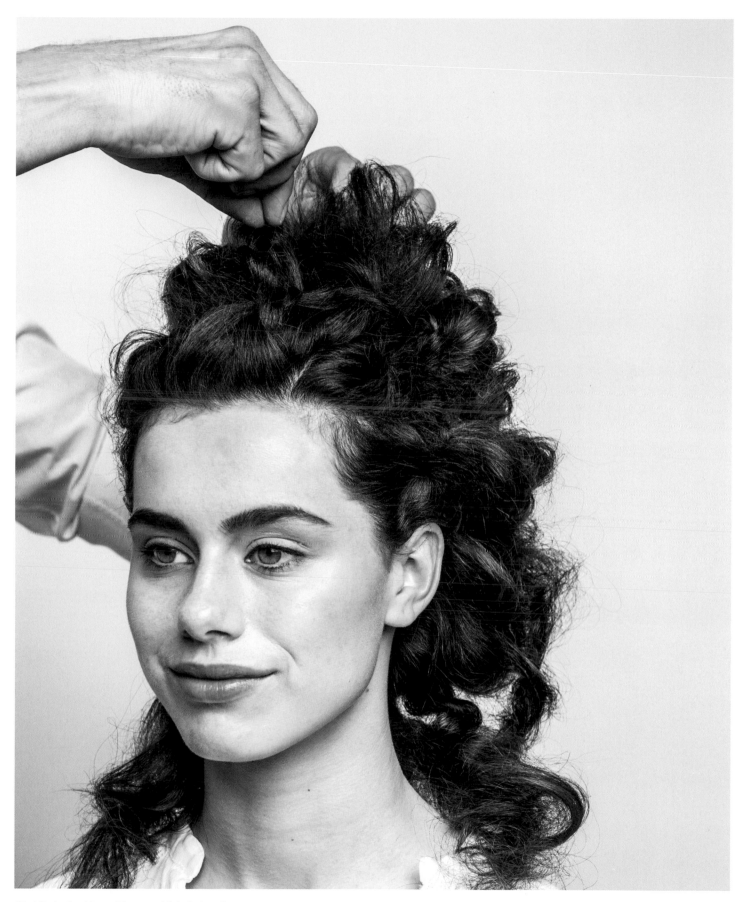

19. Lift the braids and fasten with hairpins. Set with hairspray.

Crown Braid

Messy and spontaneous, this updo is framed by a French braid.
Experiment with shape and volume to find a style that fits you!

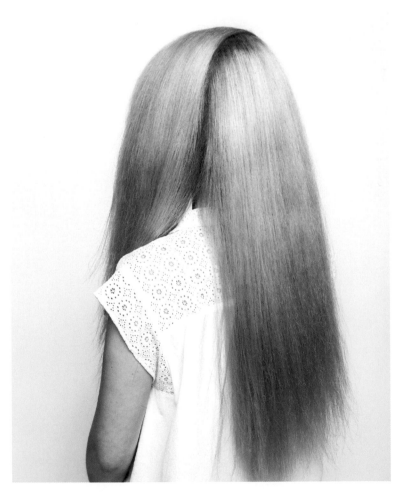

1. Divide the hair into two sections by drawing
a part from ear to ear. Brush the top section to
one side. Pull the hair in the back into a loose
ponytail. Use a fiber wax to smooth any wisps.

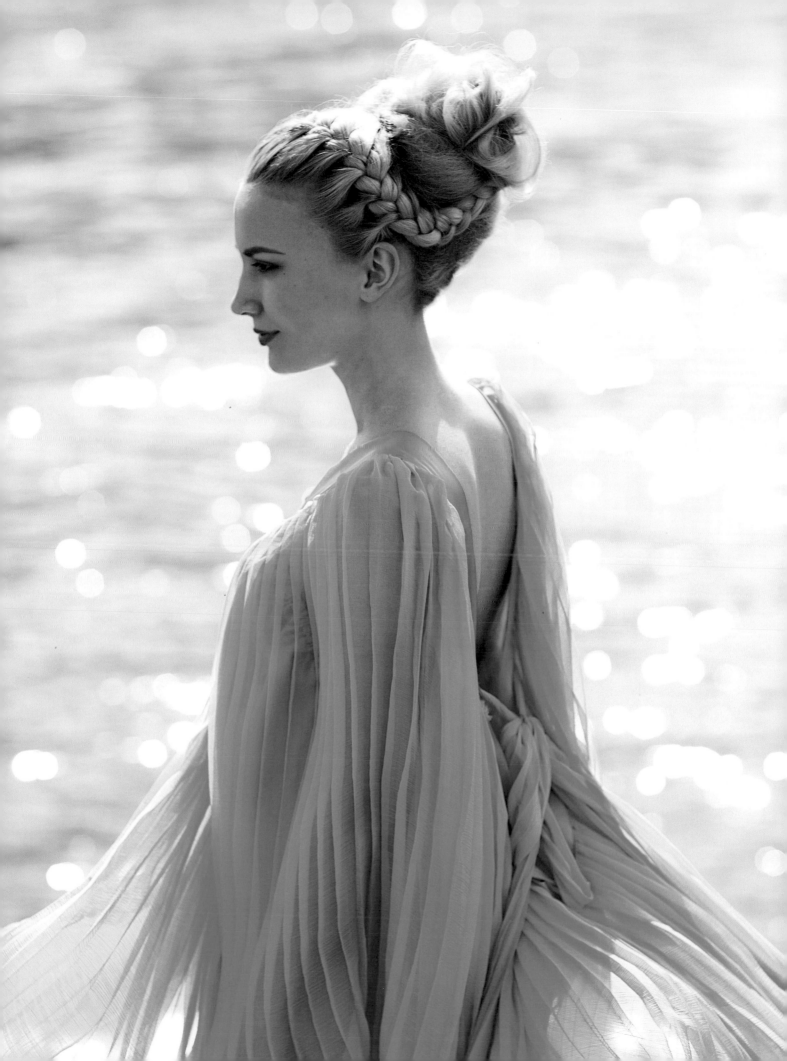

40

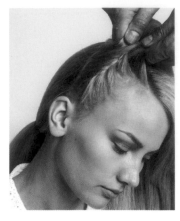 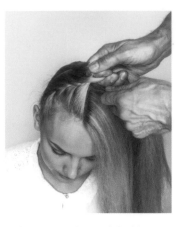 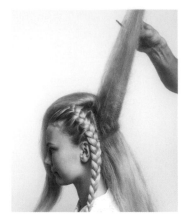 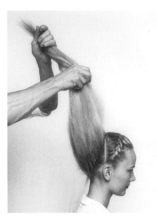

2. With the upper section of hair, make a French braid that runs from one ear to the other, then toward the shoulder. Make one round of a basic braid, where the side strands are crossed over the middle. Pick up a new strand from the outer edges with each new crossover.

3. Alternate right and left sides by taking up new strands of hair so that you add to each section. Repeat until the entire length is braided. Fasten with a small elastic. Release the lower section of hair.

4. Separate a small section of hair from the crown, about 2 inches wide. Tease the entire section.

5. Tease the rest of the hair and pull the entire section upward.

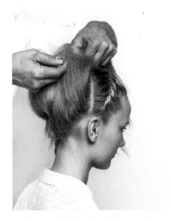 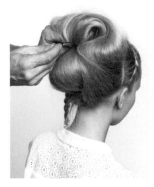

6. Fasten the hair with extra-large hairpins.

7. Fold in the ends toward the center and fasten with extra-large hairpins. The result should look spontaneous and messy. Where necessary, fasten with long hairpins. Fasten upward so that you achieve a good height for the updo.

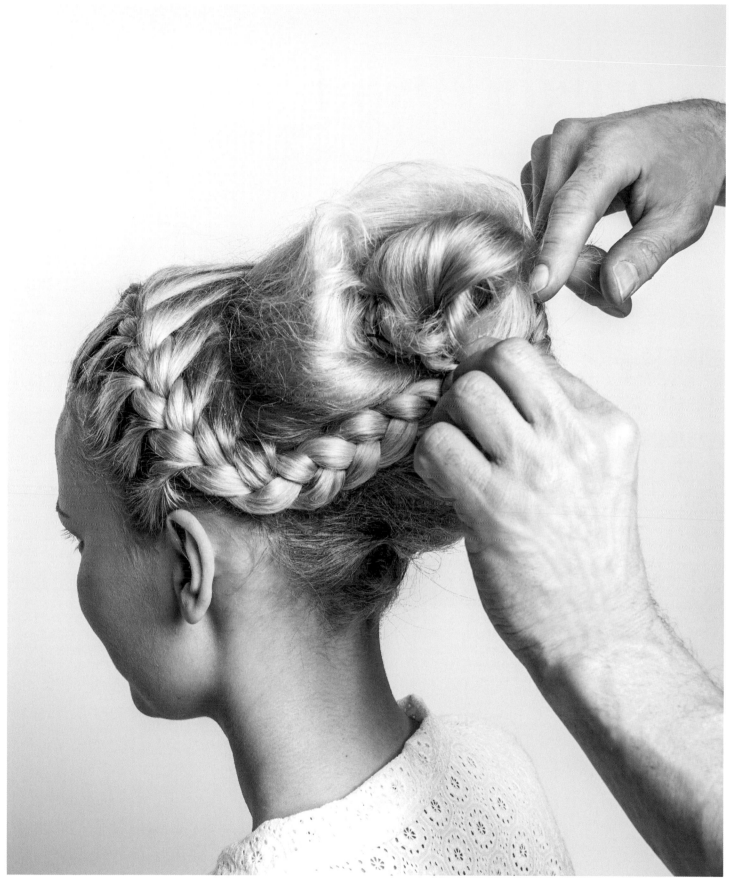

8. Add in the braid and pin it into the updo using long hairpins. Finish with hairspray.

Courtly Braid

Beautiful in its simplicity, this waterfall braid swings from the forehead, around the head, and comes to rest on the shoulder.

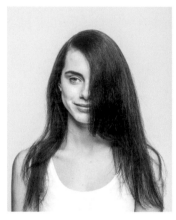 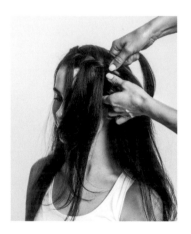 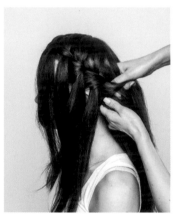 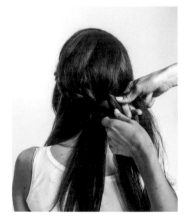

1. Make a side part. Separate a small section at the very front next to the part. Start making a three-strand braid by picking up one section of the bangs, and make one regular round.

2. For each new crossover, leave the downward-pointing strand unbraided and add in new hair to the French braid. The strands are crossed on top of one another and new hair is gathered into the braid. The strands that are left hanging free are integrated with the loose hair.

3. Continue braiding, always leaving the downward-pointing strand unbraided and picking up new hair in its place. The upper strand is filled with new hair for each crossover.

4. Braid loosely to make the braid full. Continue braiding from one side and around, finishing on the opposite side behind the ear. Braid the rest of the length and let it hang down toward the shoulder. Fasten with an elastic. Brush through the strands that are hanging down from the waterfall braid. Set with hairspray.

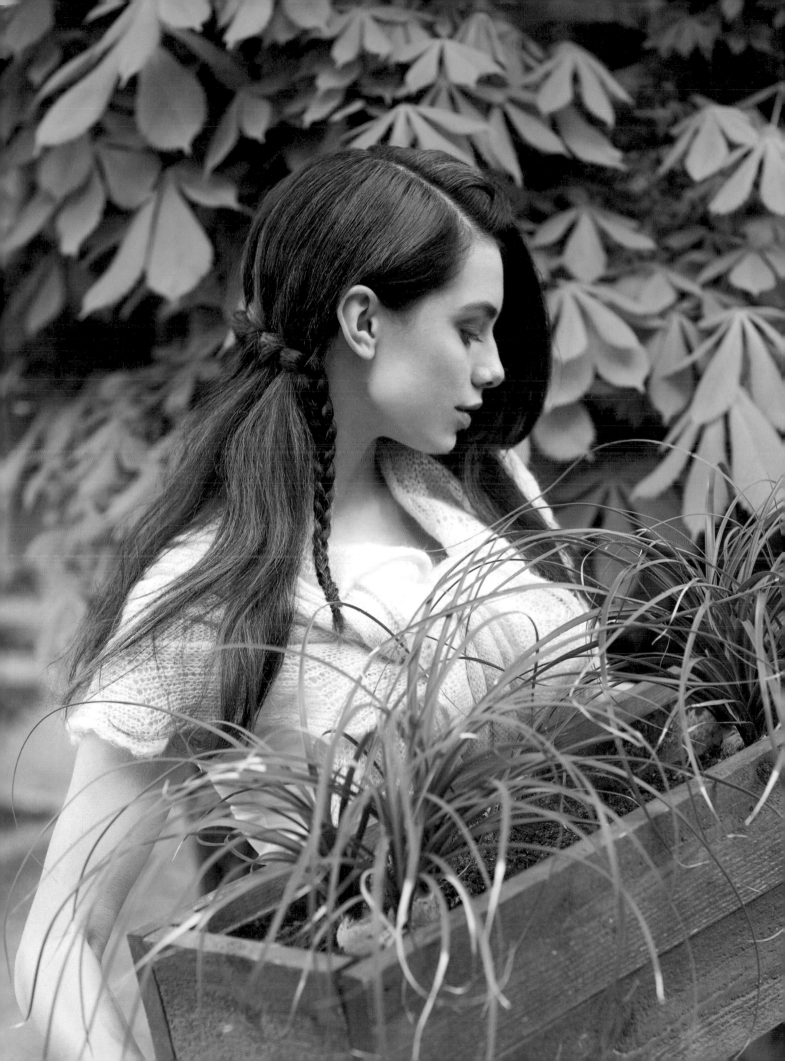

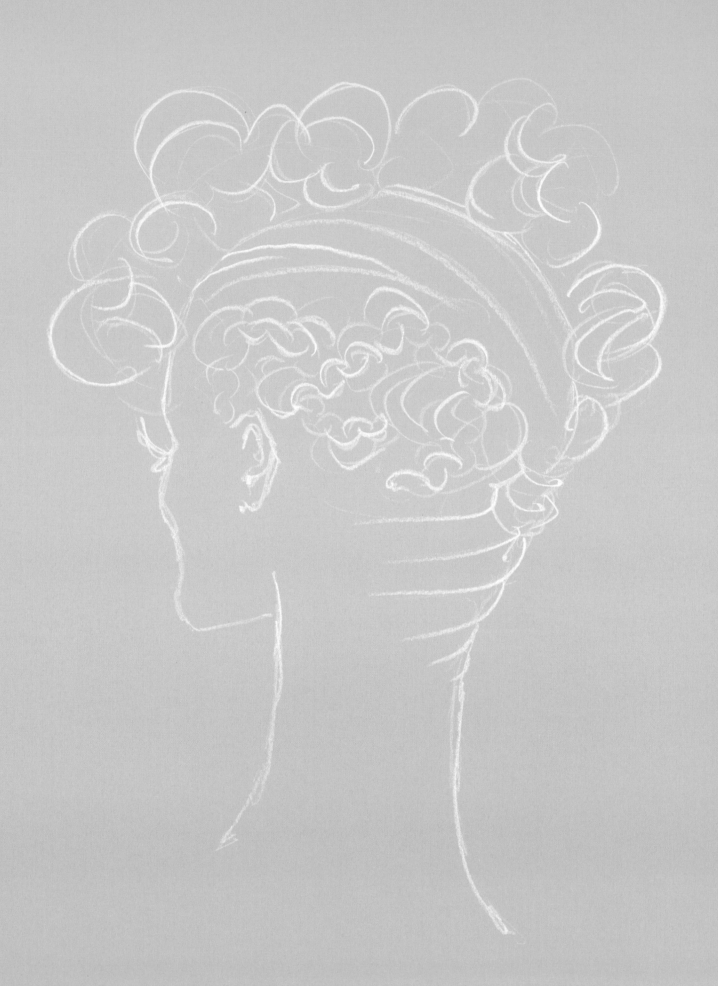

Dutch Braids

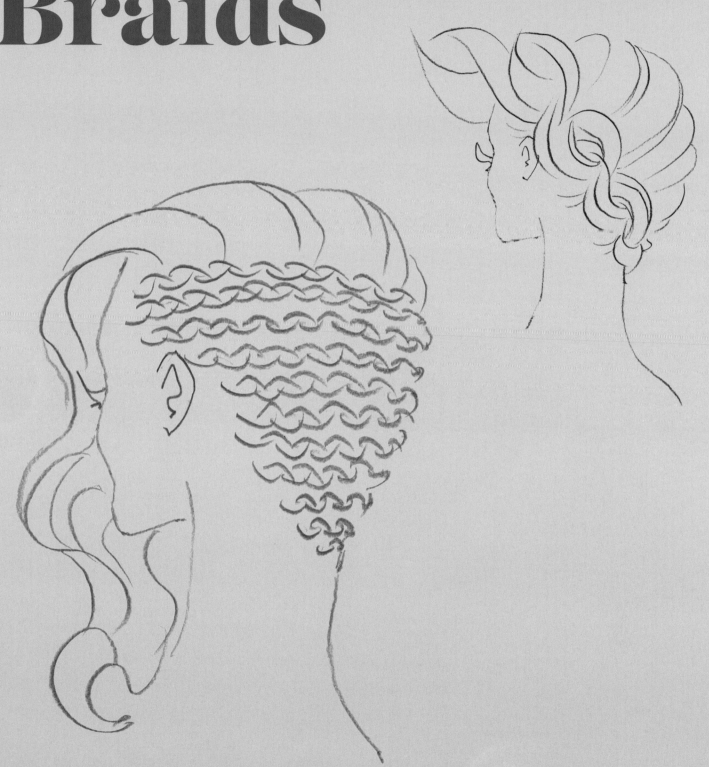

Peasant Braid

A simple hairstyle with two Dutch braids that frame the face, this goes just as well with a summer dress as with a leather jacket.

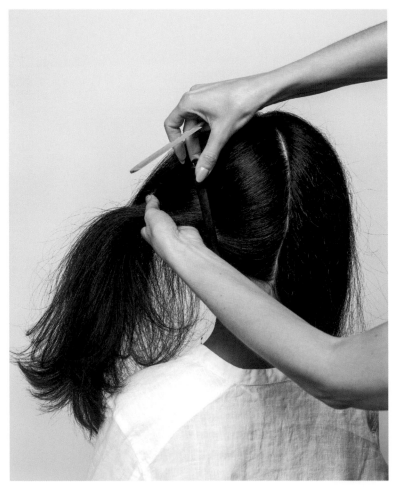

1. Divide the hair into two sections by making a straight center part all the way down to the nape of the neck. Fasten one section with a hair clip.

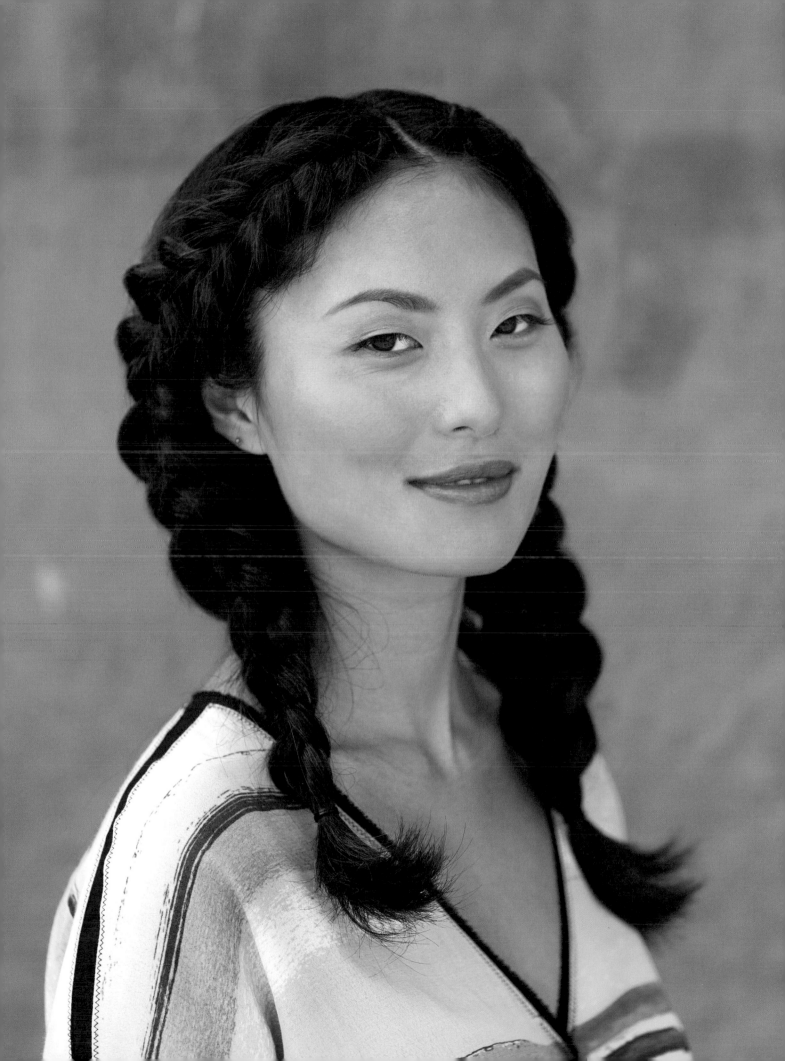

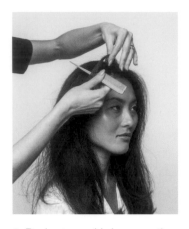

2. Begin at one side by separating out a small section of the bangs, about half an inch wide, closest to the center part.

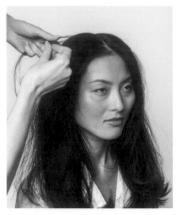

3. Make a reverse French braid. Divide the section into three strands. Make one round of a basic braid where the side strands are pulled under the center strand. Add in a new strand from the outer edges with each new crossing.

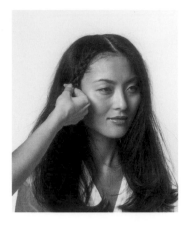

4. Alternate right and left sides by taking up new strands of hair so that you add to each section of hair. After a few rounds you will have a braid that seems to lie on top of the hair.

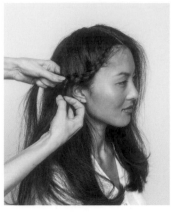

5. Braid as close to the head as possible and follow the hairline as you braid. The braid will then go around the ear and down toward the front of the neck. Repeat until the entire length is braided. Fasten with an elastic.

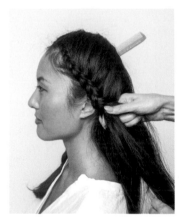

6. Repeat step 3 again on the other side of the head.

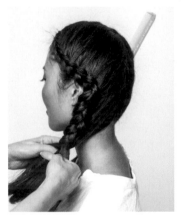

7. Braid close to the head, down toward the neck, and fasten with an elastic.

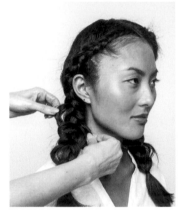

8. Create more dimension in the braid by pulling at the hair on the outside edges of the braid. Work upward and pull carefully until you achieve the feel that you want.

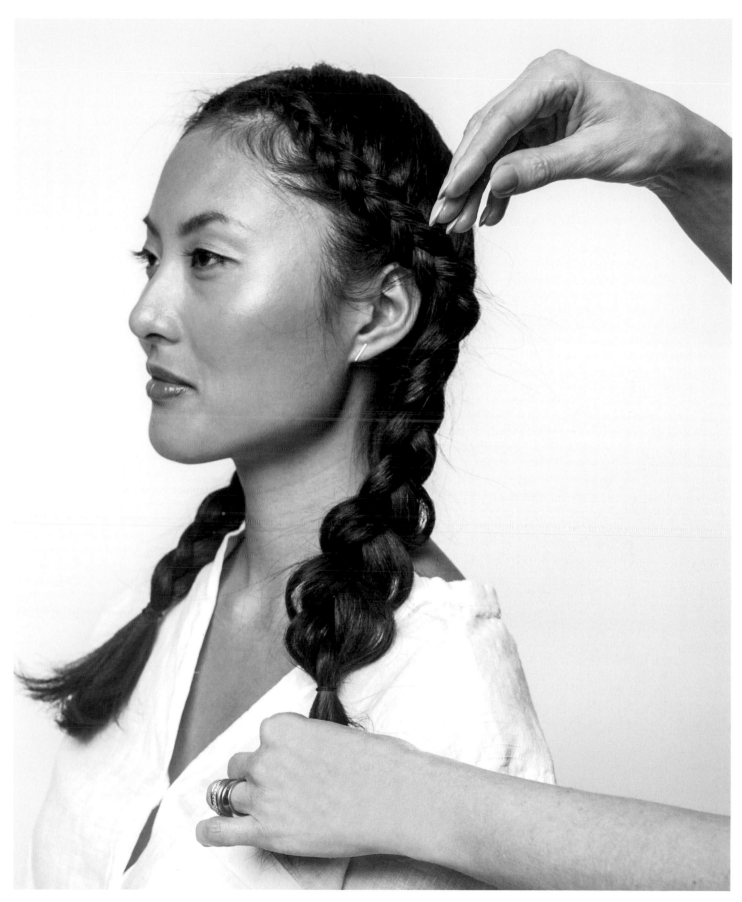

9. Fasten the upper part of the braid with hair-pins for stability, using two on each side. Rotate the hairpins and fasten against the scalp.

Triplet Braid

Classical with a twist! Here we braid all the hair in two Dutch braids going down the back, with a regular French braid in the middle. This is a hairstyle that works for any occasion.

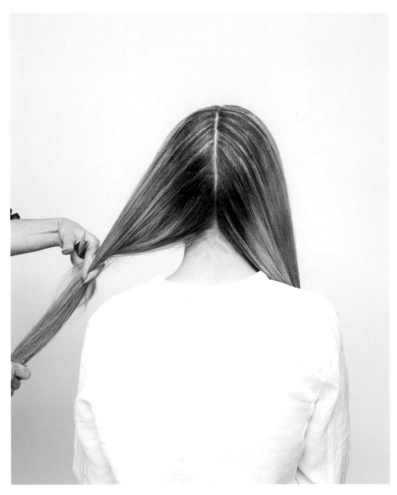

1. Make a center part down to the nape of the neck.

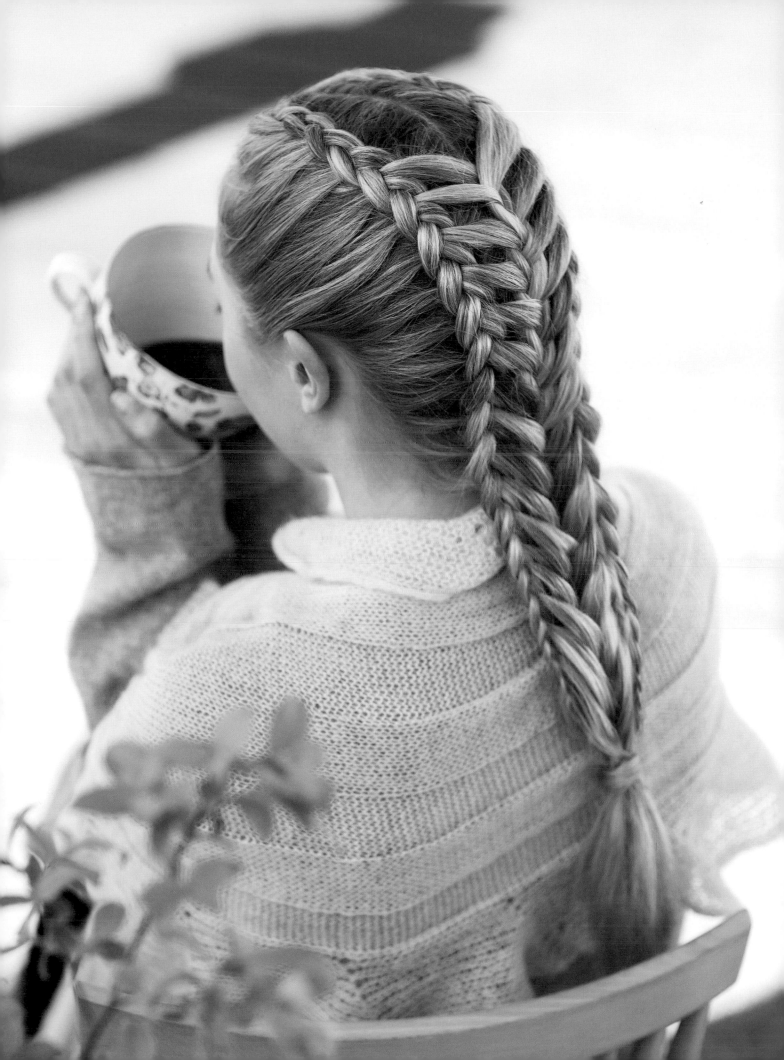

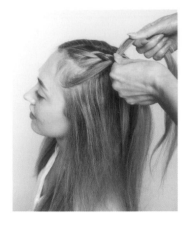

2. Begin with three strands at the front of the face, next to the center part. Make one round of a basic Dutch braid, crossing the side strands under the middle strand. Add in a new section from the outside with each new crossover.

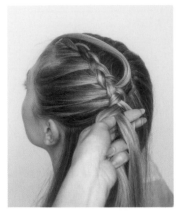

3. When you get to the curve of the head, take out one strand closest to the bottom and reserve it for later. Continue braiding as usual, but for each crossing, take out a strand nearest the bottom and set it aside until later.

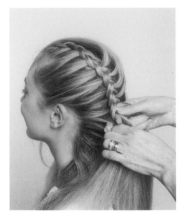

4. Alternate right and left sides by picking up new strands of hair, but set aside the one nearest the center for later. Continue until the entire length is braided.

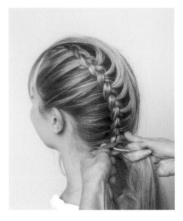

5. Continue braiding the length but reserve a strand for each cross-over, as in step 3.

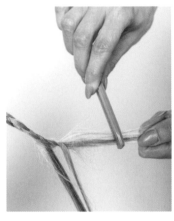

6. At the end of the braid, tease the ends.

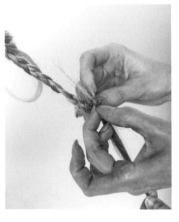

7. Make a knot to secure the braid.

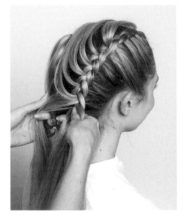

8. Repeat the same braid on the other side of the head. Braid with the same technique as in step 2. When you reach the crown, continue to braid in the same way as in step 3.

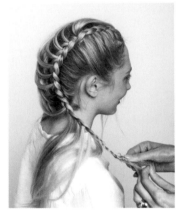

9. At the end of the braid, tease the ends and wrap around the length. Make a knot to secure the braid.

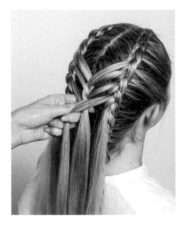

10. Gather the loose strands between the two braids and comb through them. Make a French braid using the hair between the two braids. Make one round of a basic braid, crossing the outer strands over the center strand. Then add in a new strand of hair from the side for each crossover.

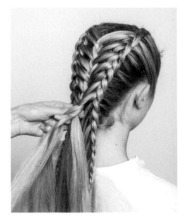

11. Alternate right and left sides by adding in new strands so that each section of hair is replenished. Repeat.

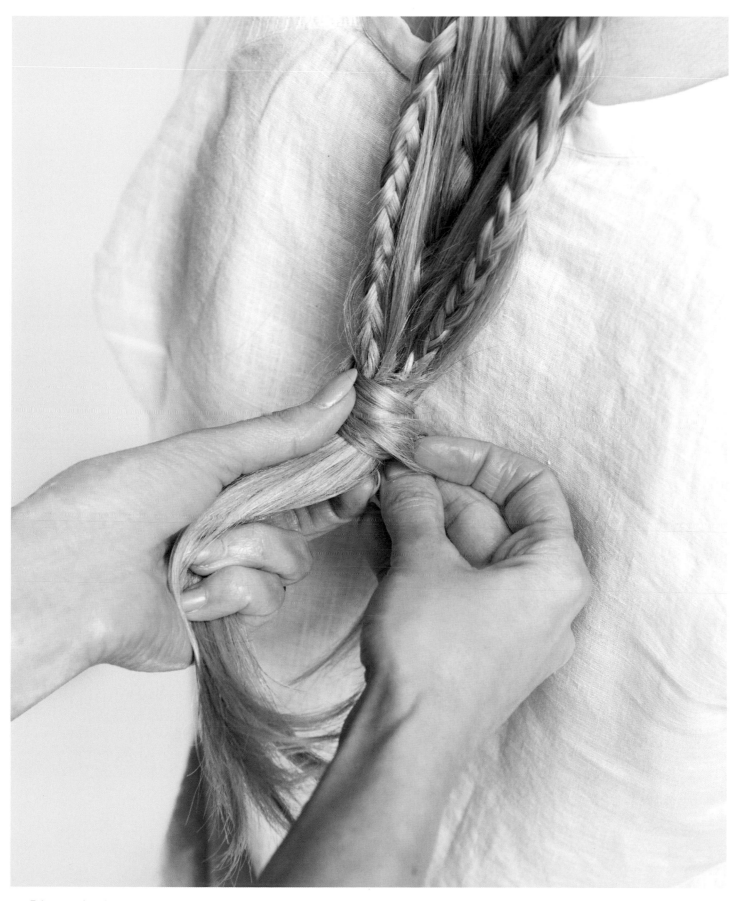

12. Bring together the ends of the other two braids into the center braid. Fasten with an elastic. Wrap a strand of hair around the elastic to conceal it. Tie a knot. Finish with hairspray.

Dutch Crown

Two Dutch braids form a wreath on top of the head. Here we leave loose strands outside the braid in order to create a unique hairstyle.

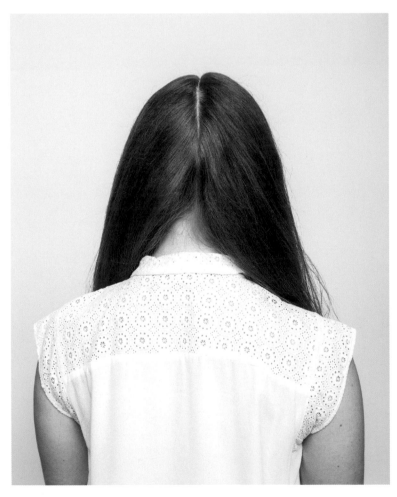

1. Divide the hair into two equal sections by drawing a center part from the forehead down to the nape of the neck.

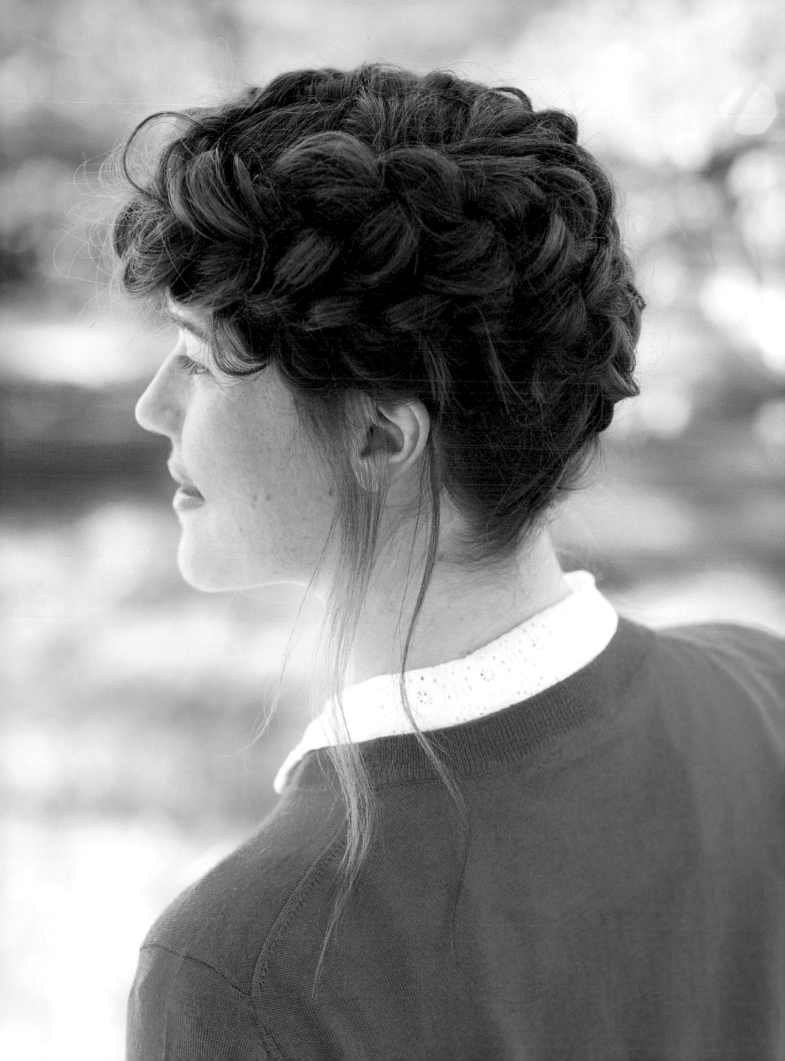

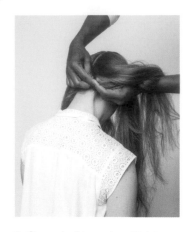
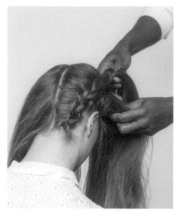
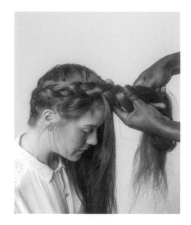
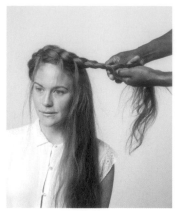

2. On each side, make a Dutch braid that runs from the nape of the neck up toward the forehead. Divide the section into three strands. Make one round of a basic braid, where the strands are crossed under the center strands. Add in a new section from the outside edges with each new crossover.

3. Alternate right and left sides by picking up new strands of hair so that you keep adding to each section.

4. Continue with the Dutch braid until you have incorporated all the loose hair, and then continue with a regular three-strand braid.

5. As you braid, pull out a few strands of hair from the braid. When you are finished, fasten with an elastic.

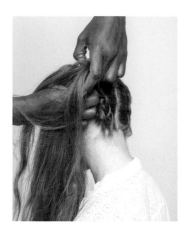
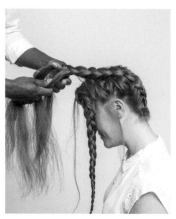
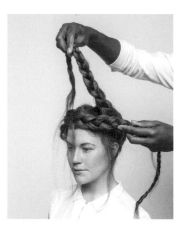
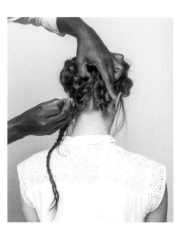

6. Now begin the other side. Braid this side as described in steps 2, 3, and 4.

7. As you braid, pull out a few strands of hair from the braid. Fasten the braid with an elastic.

8. Wrap the braids around each other and pull at them to create a more dynamic shape. The braids should form a wreath around the head.

9. Fasten the braids together with hairpins. Remember to hide the ends inside the wreath.

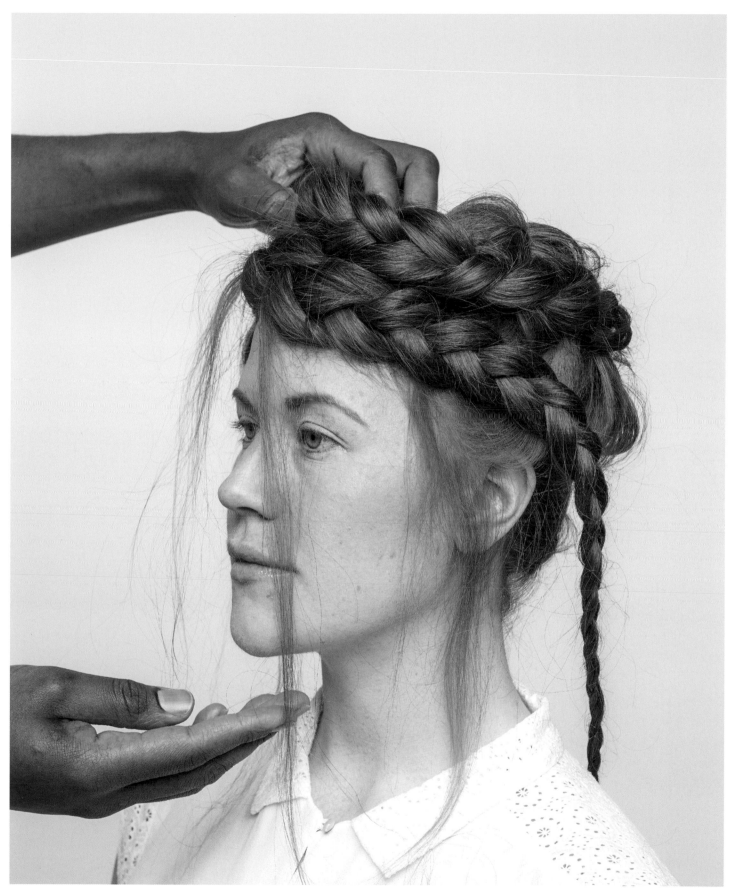

10. Leave some strands hanging outside the braid to add softness to the hairstyle. Finish with hairspray.

Stella

Soft and hard, tough and romantic, this hairstyle is all about contrasts, with thin, tight braids—or cornrows—at the neck and a pretty wave that frames the face.

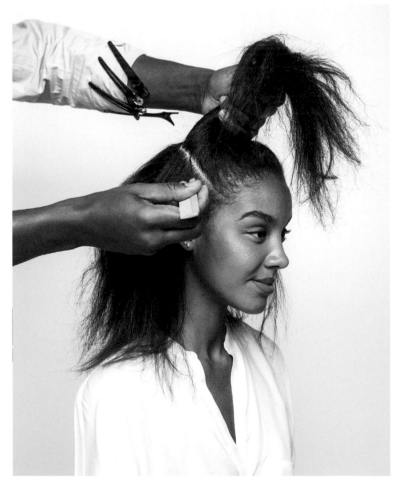

1. Divide hair into two sections, one at the crown of the head and one below. Fasten the crown section out of the way with a hair clip. You will braid the lower section of hair into several thin Dutch braids.

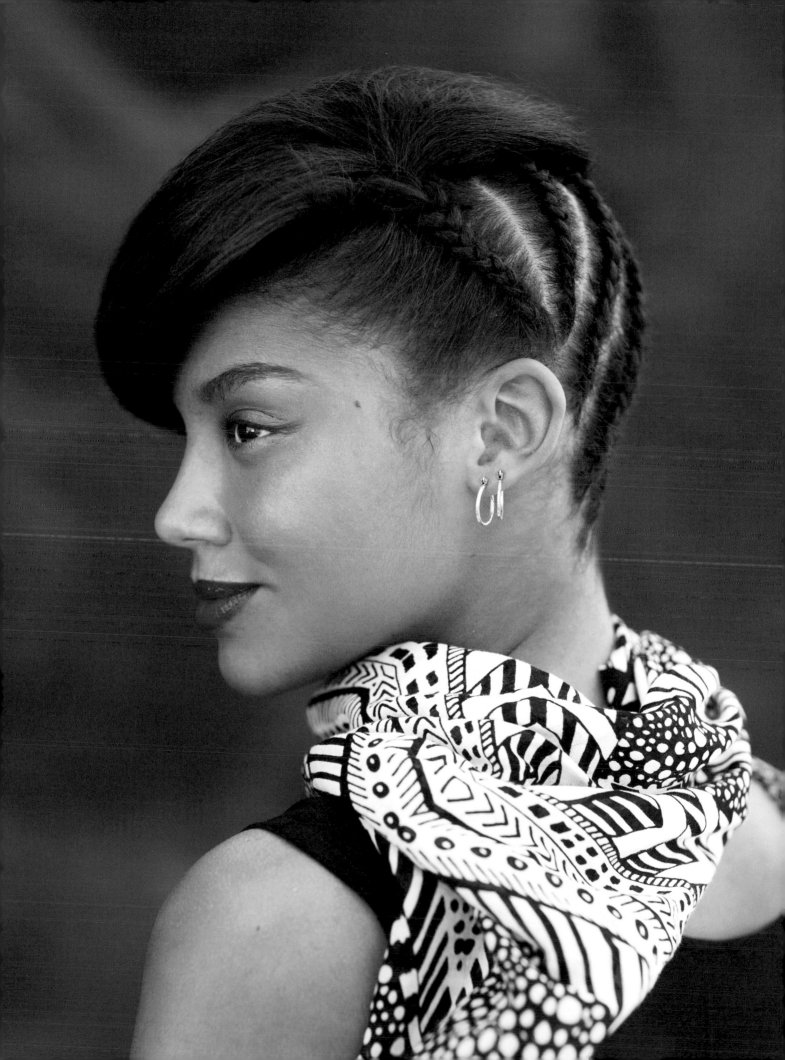

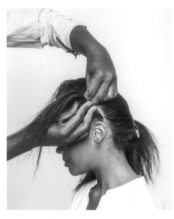

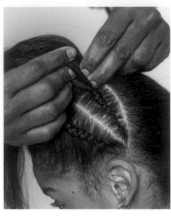

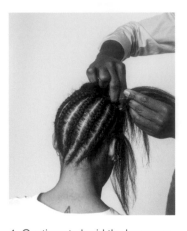

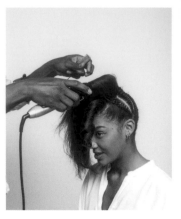

2. Separate a smaller section of hair at the ear, about 1 inch wide. Divide into three strands. Make one round of a basic braid, where the side strands are crossed under the center strand. Pick up a new strand from the outside edges with each new crossover. Alternate right and left by picking up new strands of hair and adding to each section. Braid from the bottom and as close to the head as possible, all the way to the crown hair. Fasten braid temporarily with a bobby pin.

3. Continue dividing the hair into smaller sections that you braid in the same way as in step 2.

4. Continue to braid the lower section of hair as in step 2. You can make a smaller or larger number of braids depending on what style you want. Thinner braids are easier to braid close to the head, but you can also choose to make thicker braids for a more bohemian look.

5. When you are done with the braids, gather the hair forward, toward the face.

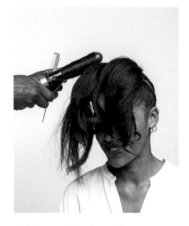

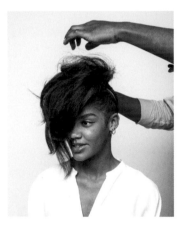

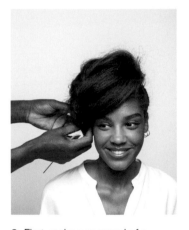

6. Use a curling iron, about 1.25 inches in diameter, to create large curls that fall down toward the eyes.

7. Gather all the hair on one side to make a loose French braid with the crown hair. Divide this section into three parts.

8. First, make one round of a basic braid, where the strands are crossed over the center strand. After the first round, add in a new strand of hair from the outside every time you make a new crossing. Alternate right and left sides by taking up new strands of hair and adding to each section. Repeat until the entire length is braided.

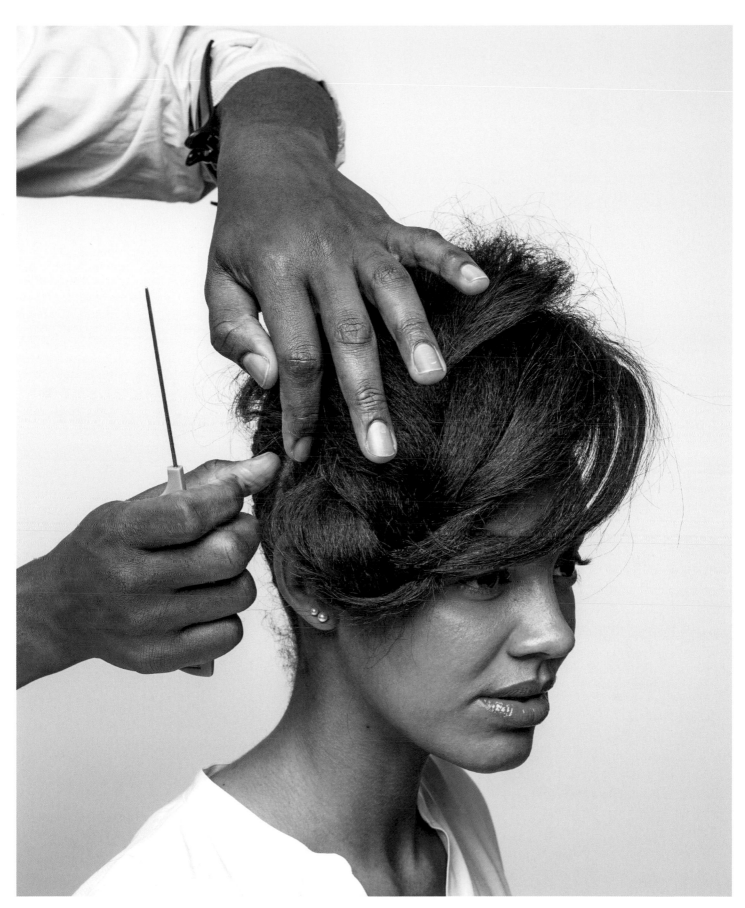

9. Now turn the ends upward and secure with a hairpin. Take out the bobby pins that you used to fasten the smaller braids and replace them with short hairpins. Pull at the braid for a softer feel. Finish with hairspray.

Coco

Tight braids matched with a playful French twist makes for a modern hairstyle that's perfect for any party!

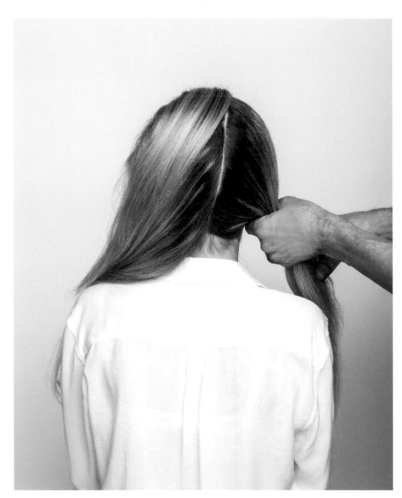

1. Divide the hair into two sections by drawing a straight center part. Put up one section in a loose ponytail.

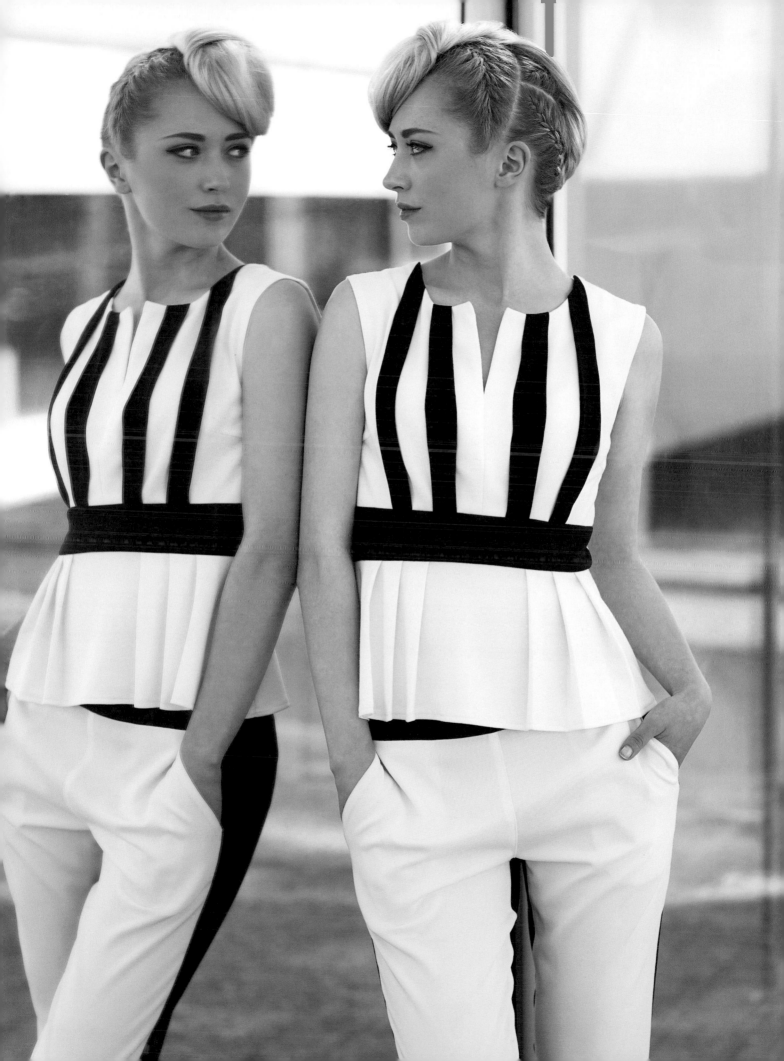

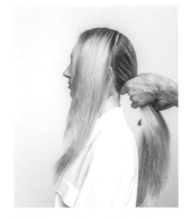

2. Begin working with the other section by drawing a part diagonally from the crown and down toward the ear, using a rattail comb. Put the rest of the hair in a ponytail as you work your way through.

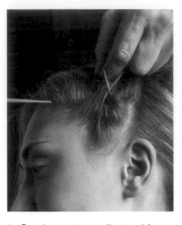

3. Section out a small strand from the very front and divide it into three sections. Now you will make a French braid. First make one round of a basic braid, where the side strands are crossed over the center strand.

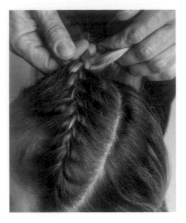

4. After the first round, pick up a new strand from the outside edges each time you make a new cross-over. Alternate right and left sides, picking up new strands each time and adding them in.

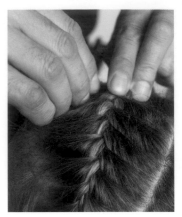

5. Braid close to the head, pulling the hair upward as you work. When you reach the end of the section, leave the remaining length unbraided. Fasten with a thin elastic.

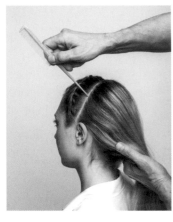

6. Now divide the rest of the hair into two sections. The part should go diagonally down toward the neck, forming a triangle.

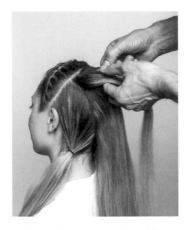

7. Fasten the front section with an elastic. Now begin working with the back section. Take a small section from the top and divide into three strands. Repeat step 4 to make a French braid here as well.

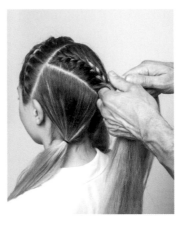

8. Keep braiding downward so that the braid lies flat against the head and doesn't lift up too much.

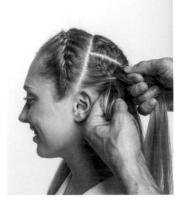

9. Now also braid the front section in the same way as in step 4. Braid toward the neck, close to the head, as before.

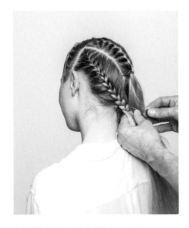

10. Continue braiding until you reach the end of the section. Fasten with a thin elastic and a bobby pin at each end.

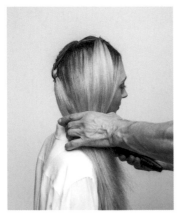

11. Gather the rest of the hair at one side of the head.

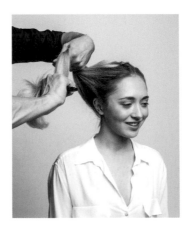

12. Take the hair in your hands and pull it diagonally upward. Twist the hair into a French twist on top of the head. Fasten with hairpins.

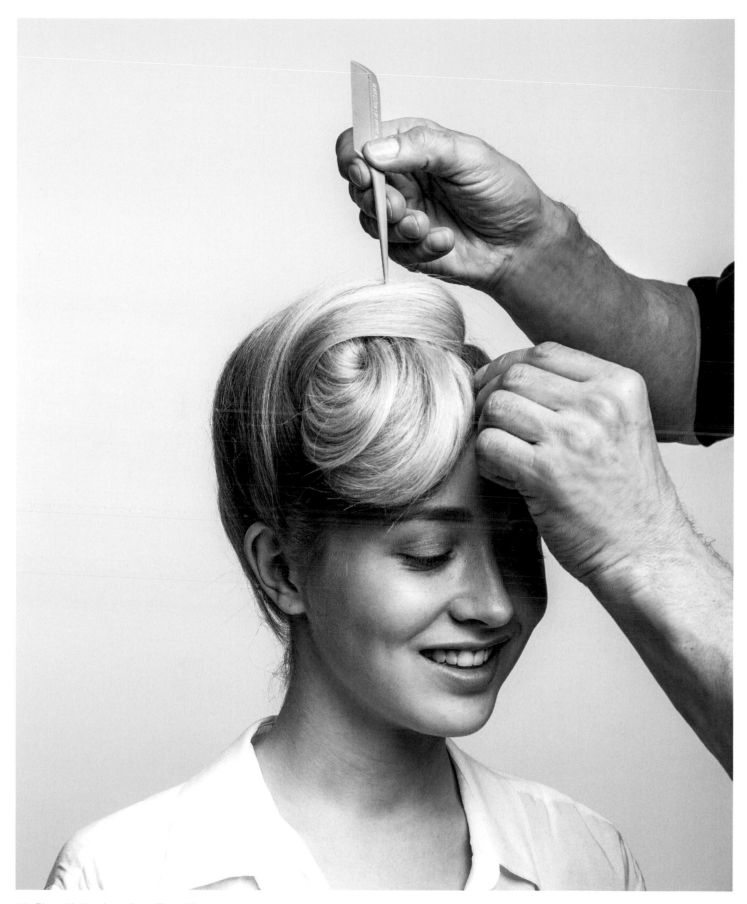

13. Play with the shape by pulling with your fingers. Secure with more hairpins if needed. Finish with hairspray.

Sidecut

Thin braids collect the hair into a pretty wave that sweeps over one shoulder. Elegance with attitude!

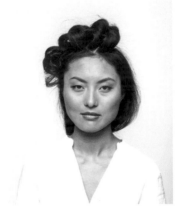

1. Curl the hair on the crown with a curling iron or heated rollers. Fasten the curls with bobby pins so that they keep their shape while you continue with the rest of the style.

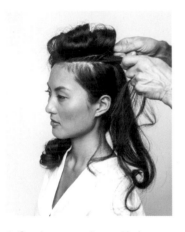

2. Section out a piece of hair about half an inch wide, running from the hairline to the back of the head. Divide the section in two, to make a French rope braid. Always twist the right part inward. Switch sides by crossing the left section over the right section, adding in a strand of remaining loose hair and twisting inward. Continue until a rope-shaped braid forms.

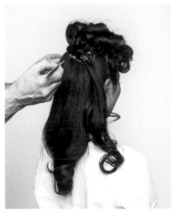

3. When you have braided just past the center of the head, fasten with a thin elastic.

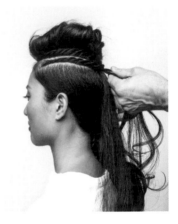

4. Now section out a new piece of hair that is the same size as the first one. Repeat the French rope braid as in steps 2 and 3.

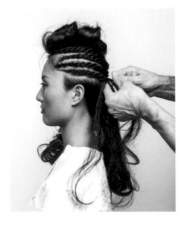

5. Repeat steps 2 and 3 until all the hair is braided.

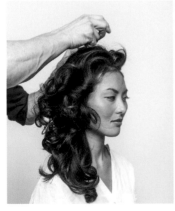

6. When all the hair is braided, remove the bobby pins from the curls at the crown.

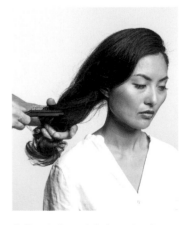

7. Brush through hair so that it forms a pretty wave on one side of the face. Finish with hairspray.

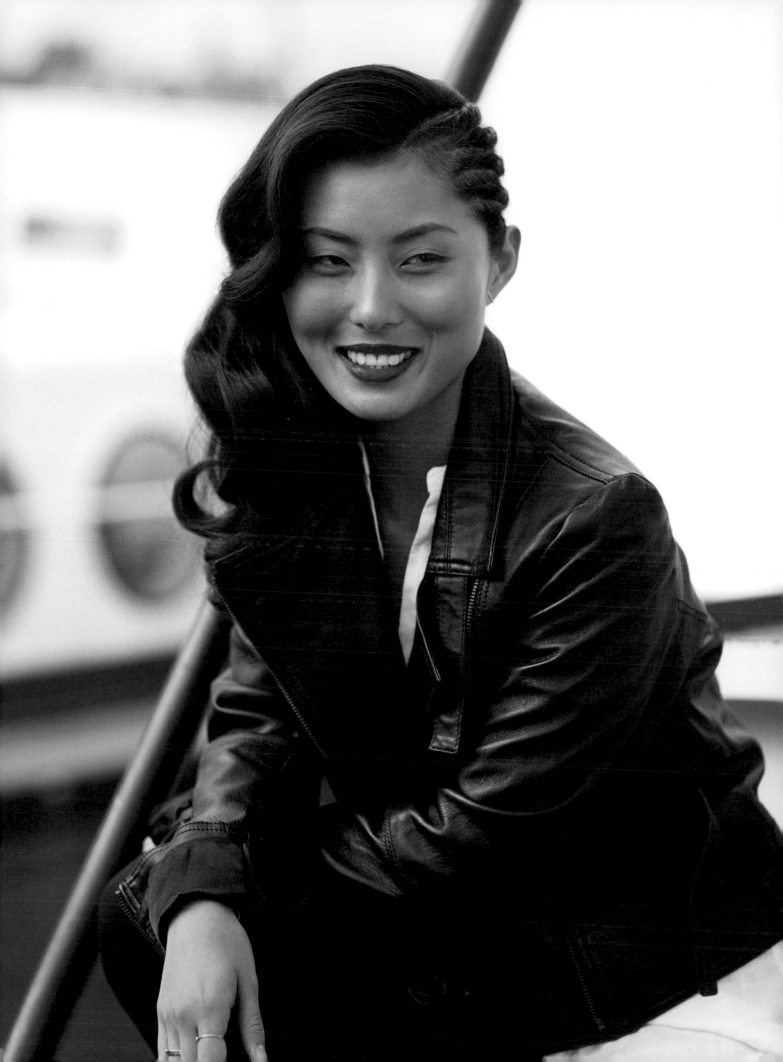

Jungle Braid

A Dutch braid looks as if it lies on top of the head, and here we use many of them for maximum impact. A fascinating hairstyle!

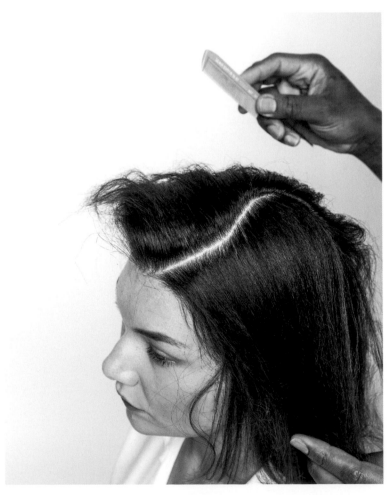

1. Separate the crown hair by drawing two wave-shaped parts using a rattail comb.

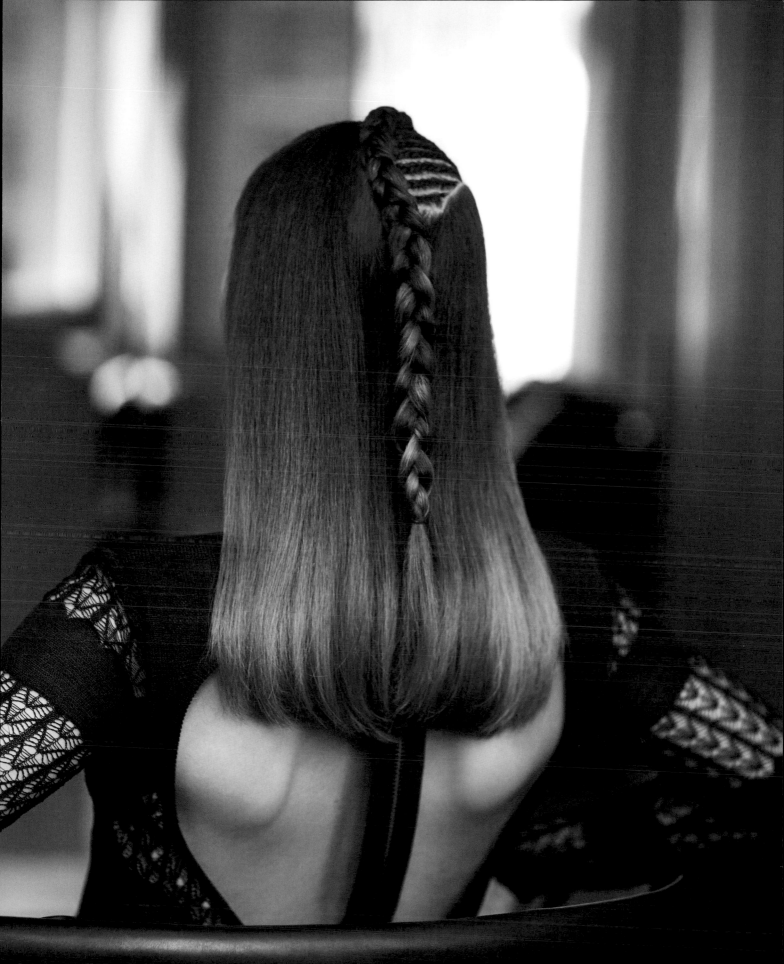

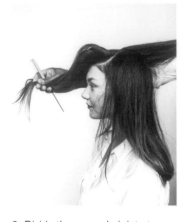

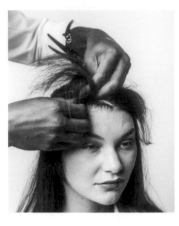

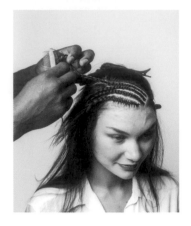

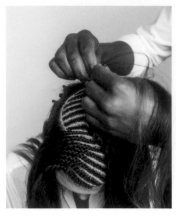

2. Divide the crown hair into two sections, one in the front and one at the back. You will begin by braiding the front section. This hairstyle consists of several small Dutch braids.

3. Section out a small piece of hair at the very front by the hairline. Divide piece into three strands. Make one round of a basic braid, where the side strands are crossed under the center strand. Then take up a new strand from the outside edges each time you make a new crossover. Alternate right and left sides by taking up new strands of hair, adding to each section of hair.

4. After a few crossings you will have a braid that looks like it is lying on top of the hair. Braid tightly against the head, moving away from the face. Leave 4 inches of the length unbraided. Continue braiding the front part of the hair in small sections about half an inch wide. Use the same technique as in step 3.

5. Now braid the rear section in the opposite direction, in small rows about half an inch wide. Use the same technique as described in steps 3 and 4.

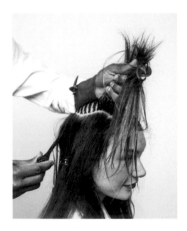

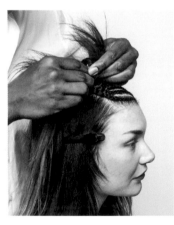

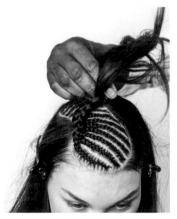

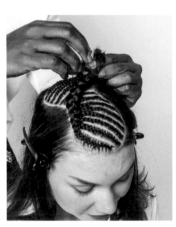

6. Return to the front section and turn the ends upward.

7. Beginning at the first braid, make a Dutch braid with the unbraided ends of the small braids, using the same technique as described in steps 3 and 4.

8. Continue braiding. The braid should curve through the braided rows of hair and meet the ends of the rear section.

9. Integrate the ends of the rear section into the braid as well, and continue braiding down toward the neck. Fasten with an elastic.

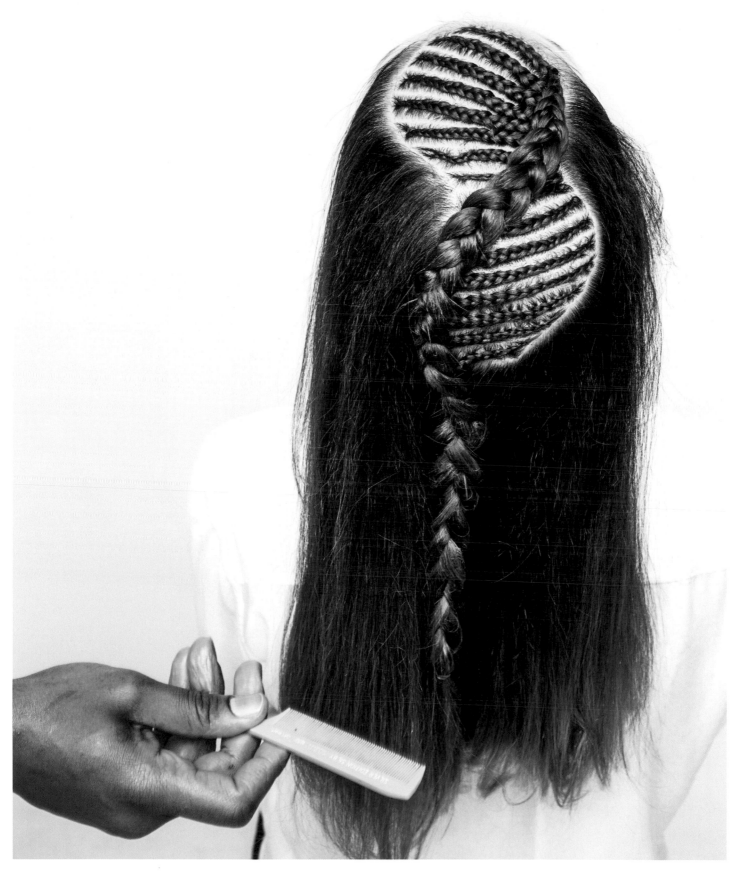

10. Let the rest of the hair hang freely. You might want to use a straightening iron to create a smooth surface. Finish with a light hairspray.

Star Braid

In this updo, we alternate Dutch braids with rope braids that form cornrows. These are all gathered into a high-impact knot on top of the head.

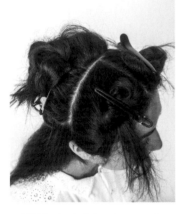 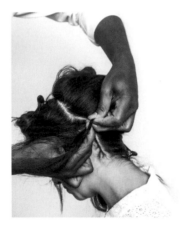 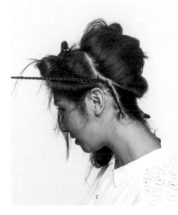 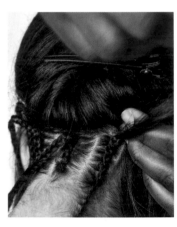

1. Divide the hair into four sections by first drawing a part from ear to ear. Then divide the crown hair with a center part. Divide the rear hair into two sections, one upper and one lower.

2. Begin braiding the lowest section, making Dutch braids. Section out a small piece at the ear and divide it into three strands. Braid upward, staying close to the head. First make one round of a basic braid, where the side strands are crossed under the center strand. After the first round, pick up a new strand from the outer edges each time you make a new crossover.

3. Repeat the technique described in step 2 until the entire length is braided. After a few crossings you will have formed a braid that looks like it is lying on top of the hair.

4. Repeat the technique described in step 2 until all the hair in the lower section is braided.

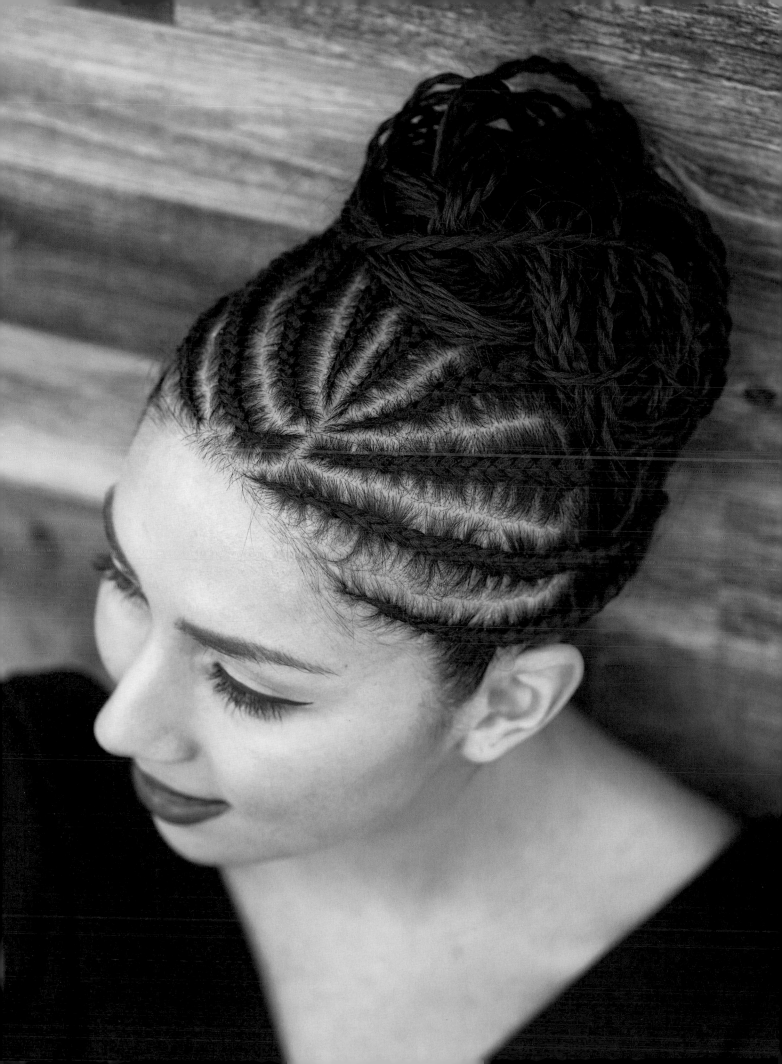

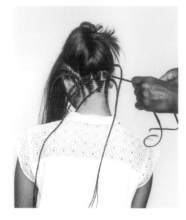

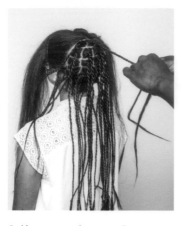

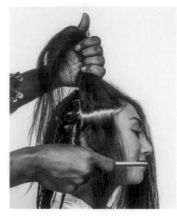

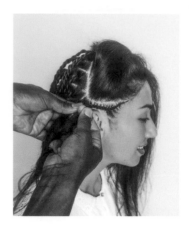

5. Continue to the midsection. Divide this hair into three smaller sections of three strands each. Now you will make rope braids. Divide each section further into two strands. Twist the right strand inward. Switch sides by twisting the left strand over the right one. Now twist the right strand inward. Switch places again and repeat so that a rope-shaped braid is formed. Braid the entire length of hair and fasten with a thin elastic.

6. Keep repeating step 5 to create a grid pattern of rope braids on the crown of the head. When the back section of the head is finished, continue on to the side sections.

7. Begin with the right side by sectioning out a piece of hair farthest down toward the ear, a little more than 1 inch wide.

8. Make a Dutch braid in the same way as in step 2. After a few crossings you will have formed a braid that looks like it is lying on top of the hair.

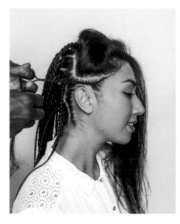

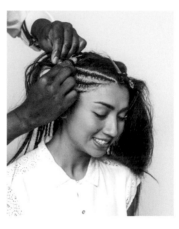

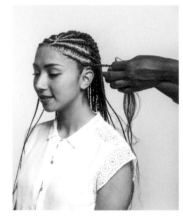

9. When you reach the end of the section, finish with a rope braid as described in step 5. Fasten with a small elastic.

10. Work your way upward. The farther up on the head you braid, the more you will curve the braids. Experiment with the shape, and feel free to let the braids be asymmetrical.

11. Repeat steps 7 to 9 until both of the front sections are braided.

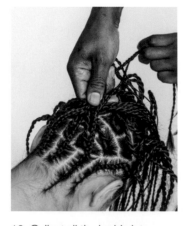

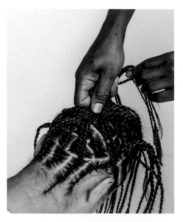

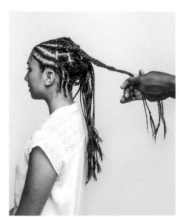

12. Collect all the braids into a Dutch braid. Bow the head down and braid from the bottom up. First make one round of a basic braid, where the side braids are crossed over the center braid.

13. Bring in one new braid from the outside edges each time you make a new crossing. Alternate right and left sides by adding in new braids so that you add to each section. Repeat until the entire length is braided. Fasten with an elastic.

14. Make two regular three-strand braids using the front braids. First cross the right braid over the center braid, and then the left braid over the center braid. Alternate right and left sides. Fasten with elastic bands.

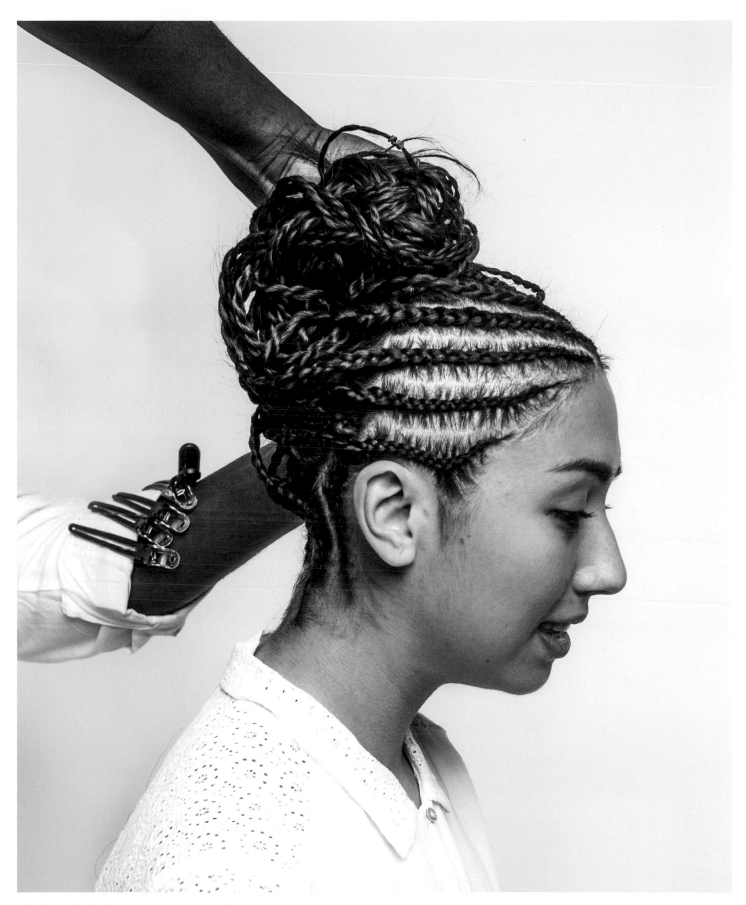

15. Fasten the braids into an updo on top of the head using long hairpins. Experiment with the shape until you find a style that you like.

Tiara Braid

Create a tiara made of braids! This style consists of two Dutch braids that end in a low bun.

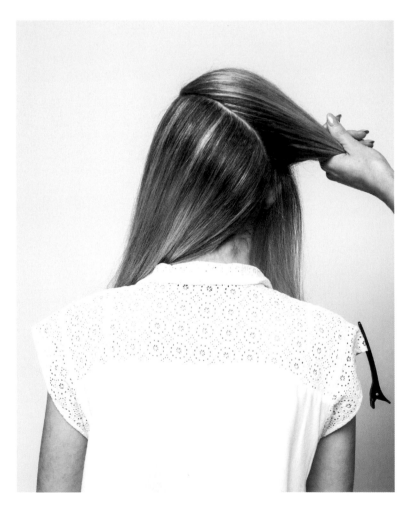

1. Make a low side part, level with the end of the eyebrow. The part goes around the head and ends at the opposite ear.

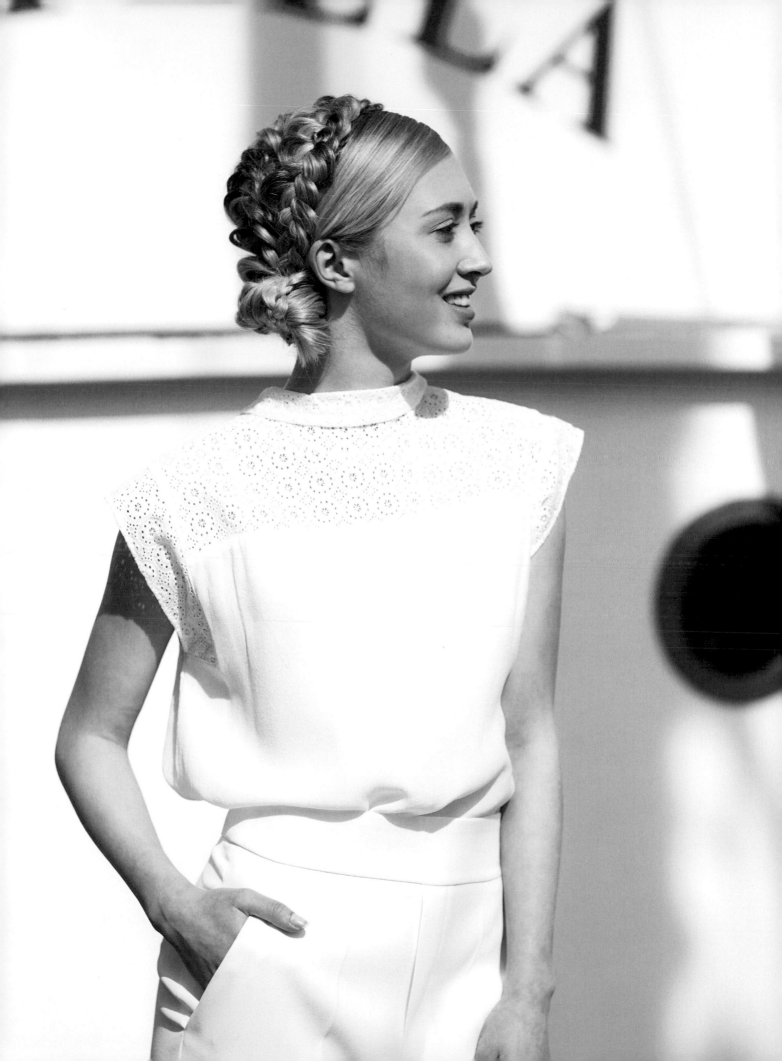

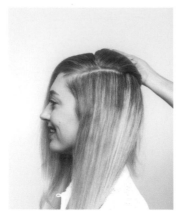

2. Separate a piece of hair at the crown, about 4 inches wide. Put up this section temporarily with a hair clip.

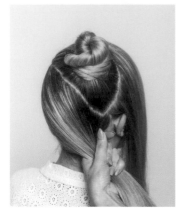

3. Pull the lowest section of hair to the side, toward one ear, and fasten in a ponytail using an elastic.

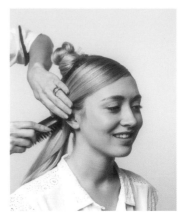

4. Comb the bang section smoothly in behind the ear. Fasten with a bobby pin.

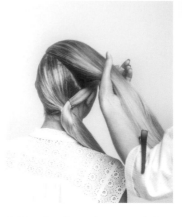

5. Now brush out the crown hair, using a light hairspray if desired to make the hair sleek. Divide into two sections.

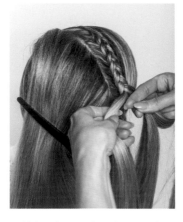

6. Using the section closer to the front, make a Dutch braid. Divide this section into three strands. Make one round of a basic braid, where the side strands are crossed under the center strand. Then pick up a new strand from the outside edges with each new crossover. For each new crossing, add in new hair so that each section is replenished. After a while you will see a braid that seems to lie on top of the hair. Fasten with an elastic.

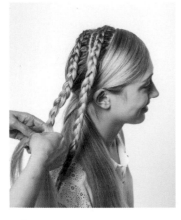

7. Continue to the other section. Repeat the braid as described in step 6. Fasten with an elastic. Make sure the braids are tight and follow the head.

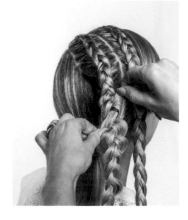

8. Pull at the braids to add texture, pulling from the bottom up.

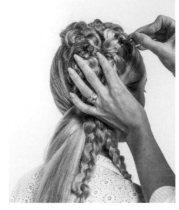

9. Lift the braids using hairpins. Rotate and fasten the braid using the pin.

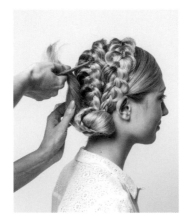

10. Twist the braids together with the ponytail and turn the ends up.

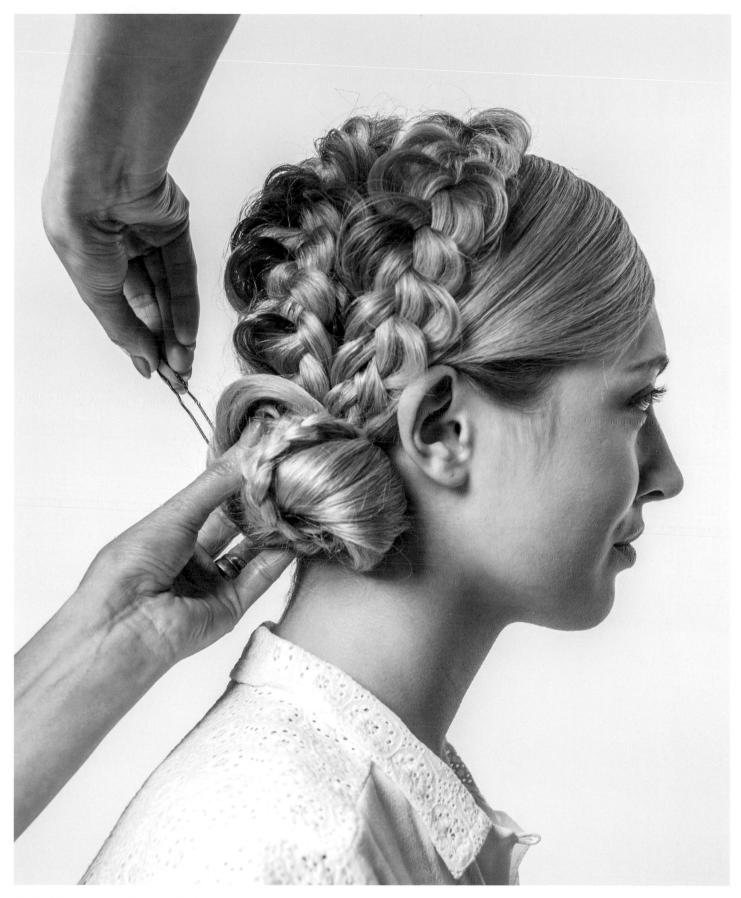

11. Tuck in the ends and fasten with short hairpins.

Wreath Braid

This hairstyle, with its half Dutch braids, offers a sweeping updo that is both playful and elegant!

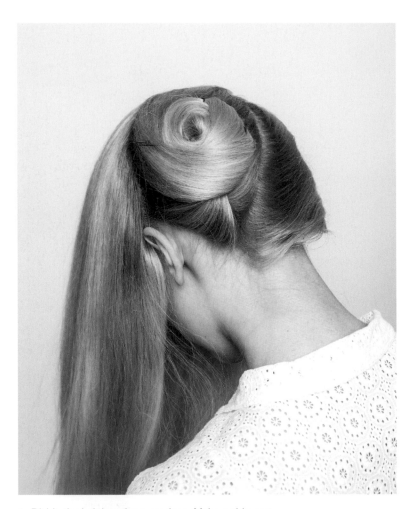

1. Divide the hair into three sections. Make a side part diagonally down toward the neck. Then make another part that runs from the side part in the middle of the crown, down toward the ear. Fasten the middle section out of the way with a hair clip.

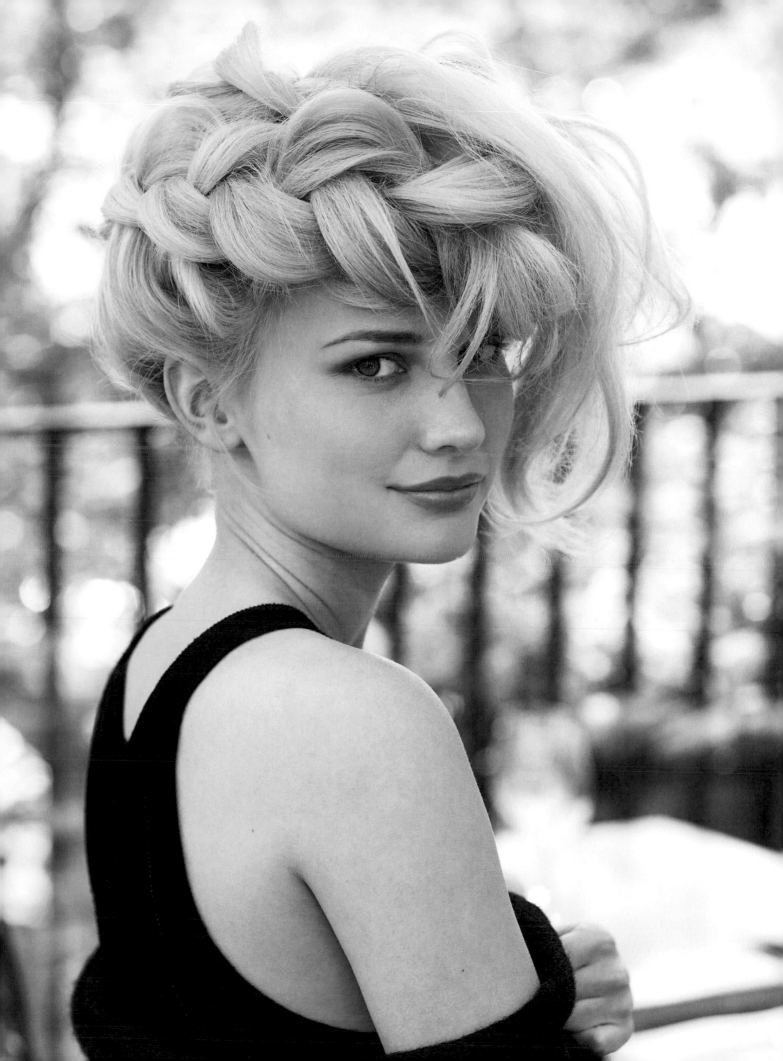

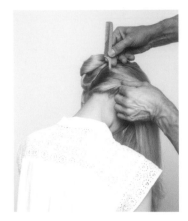

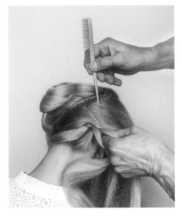

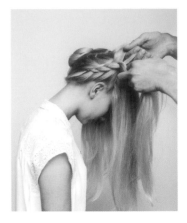

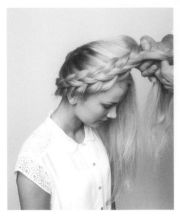

2. Begin braiding the lower section by separating out a smaller part and dividing it into three strands.

3. Begin making a half Dutch braid. First make one round of a basic braid, where the side strands are crossed under the center strand. After the first round, add in a new strand of hair from one side each time with each new crossing.

4. Continue braiding, but only add in new hair from one side.

5. The braid should go upward and alongside the head but remain loose and relaxed.

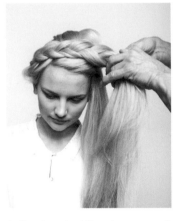

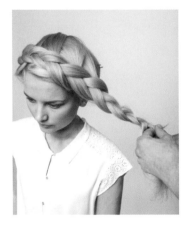

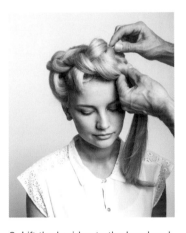

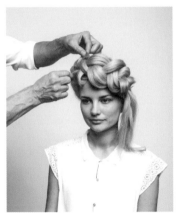

6. Continue braiding down toward the opposite ear.

7. Leave part of the length unbraided. Fasten with an elastic.

8. Lift the braid onto the head and fasten it with hairpins.

9. Pull at the braid to make it even looser.

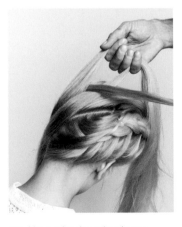

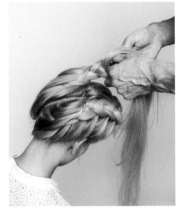

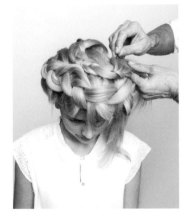

10. Now take the other lower section and brush upward. Gather the hair together. Separate one large section and divide this into three strands. Make a half Dutch braid with these strands as well.

11. Begin with one round of a basic braid, where the side strands are crossed under the center strand. Then add in a new strand of hair from one side with each new crossing. Repeat by adding in hair from the side when you braid. Leave part of the length unbraided.

12. Let the ends fall down toward the face and fasten with hairpins.

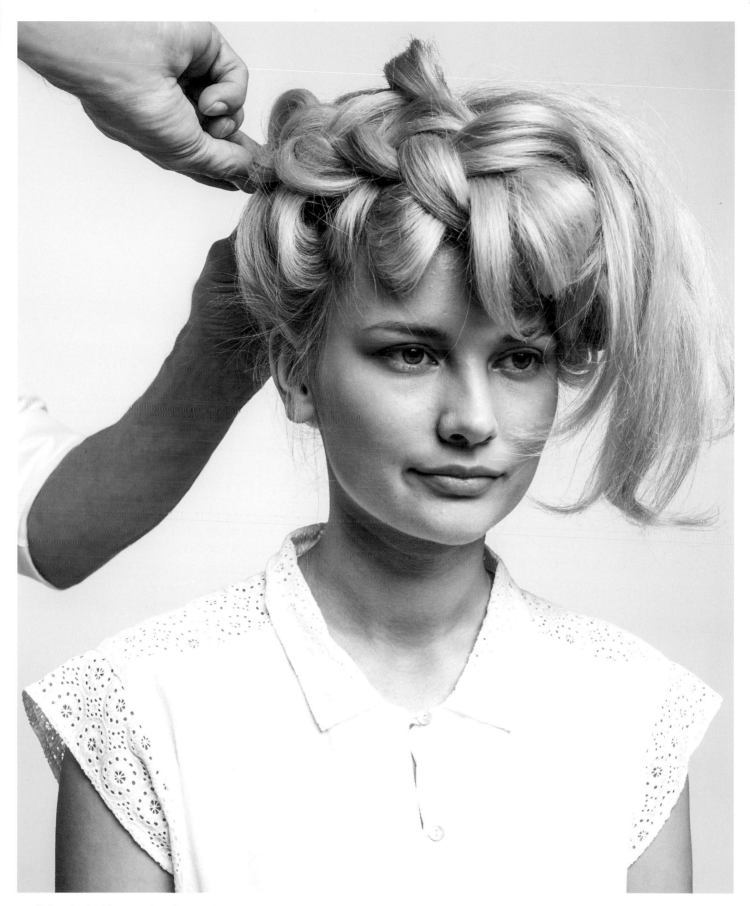

13. Pull at the braid, as much as it can tolerate without disintegrating. If there are any ends you want to get out of the way, twist them loosely and fasten into the updo.

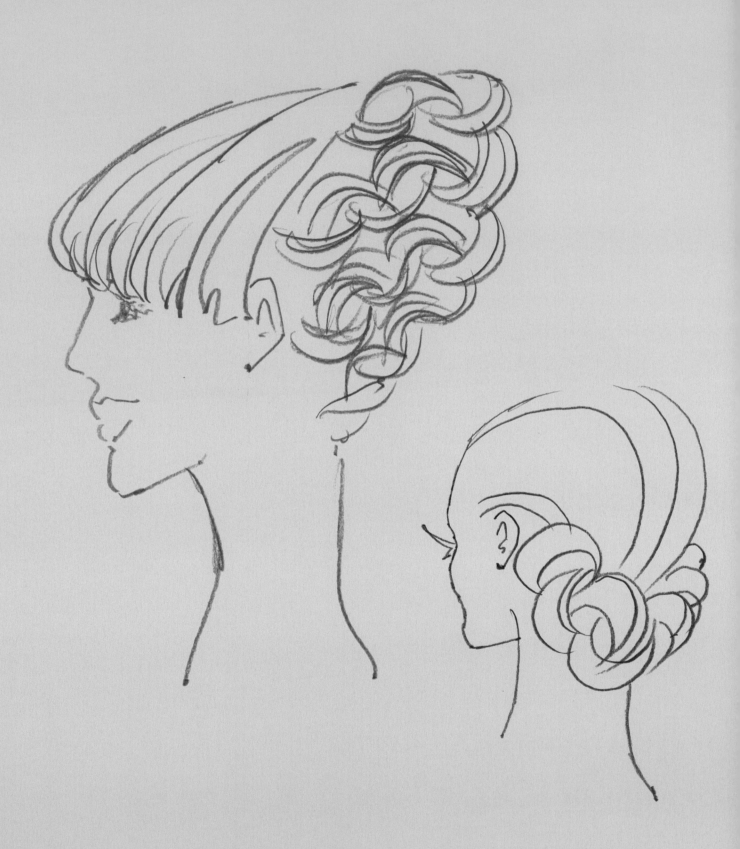

Knotted Braids and Fishtail Braids

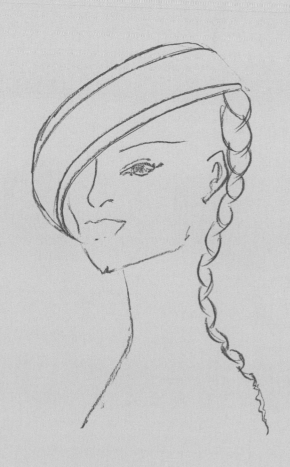

Fishtail-braided Pony

A braided hairdo does not have to be difficult or time-consuming to make. A high ponytail turns into something special when it transitions into a fishtail braid.

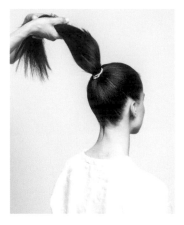

1. Gather the hair into a ponytail high up on the head. Fasten tightly using an elastic.

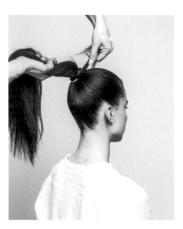

2. Take out a strand of hair from the ponytail and twist it. Wrap the twisted strand around the base of the ponytail and fasten with a hair-pin. This is a good way to conceal the elastic.

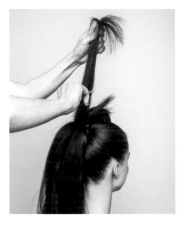

3. Divide the ponytail into three sections. Tease the midsection to create volume.

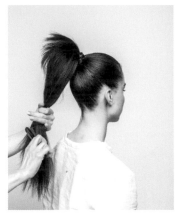

4. Gather the ponytail down so that the teasing doesn't show. Carefully brush through the ponytail.

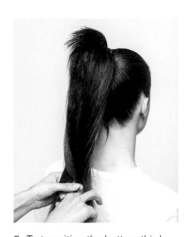

5. To transition the bottom third of the ponytail to a fishtail braid, divide the hair into two sections. Hold one section of hair in each hand. Take a small strand from the underneath side of one section.

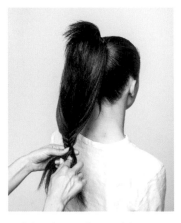

6. Bring the small strand from under the hair section around the outside edge and across to the opposite side. Alternate sides, crossing strands from one side to the other. Always have one section of hair in each hand.

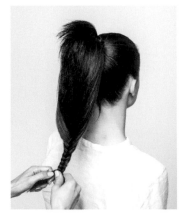

7. The thinner the strands you take from each section of hair, the more defined the fishtail pattern will be. Fasten with an elastic.

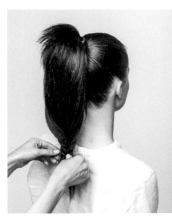

8. Pull carefully at the braid to create a more dynamic shape. Use any pieces of hair that may stick out of the braid to create your own look.

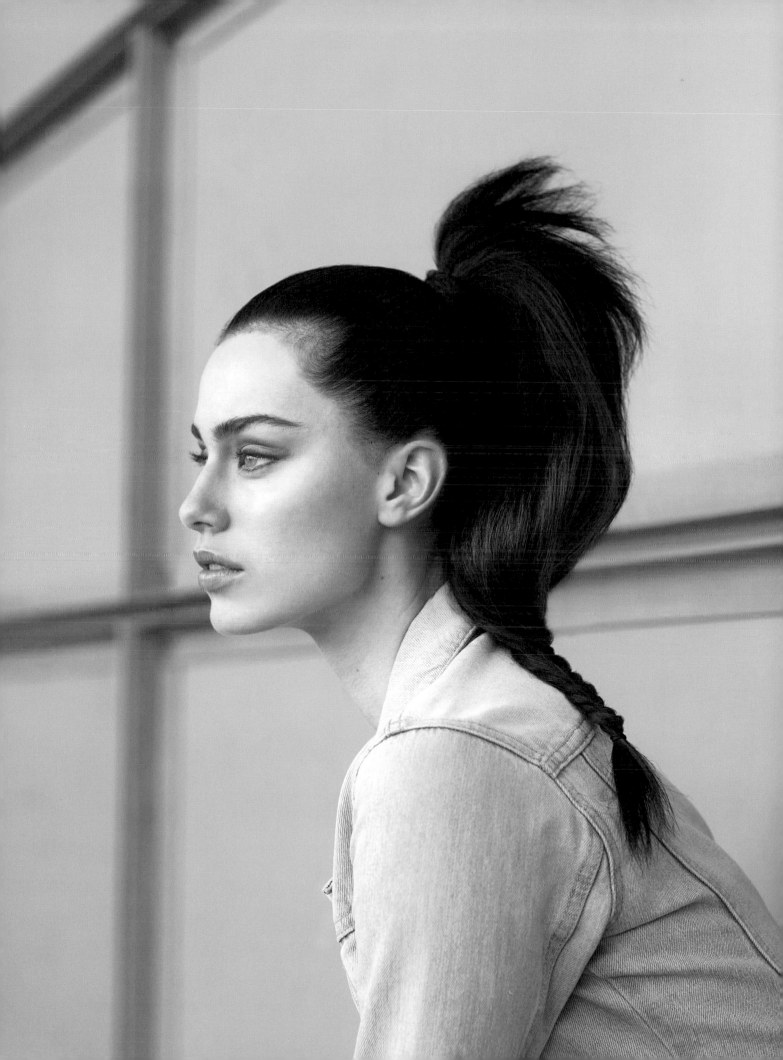

Bohemian Braid

Messy fishtail braids combined with unbraided hair, this is the hairstyle for you if you want a bohemian and relaxed look!

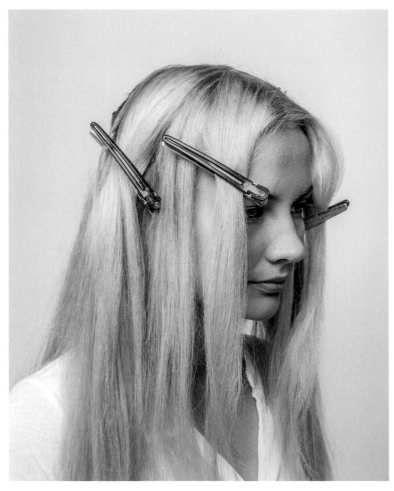

1. Brush through the hair and make a center part. Separate two sections of hair on each side of the head. The sections should be 2 inches wide with a 1-inch-wide strand in between that will remain unbraided. Clip the four sections with hair clips to keep them out of the way.

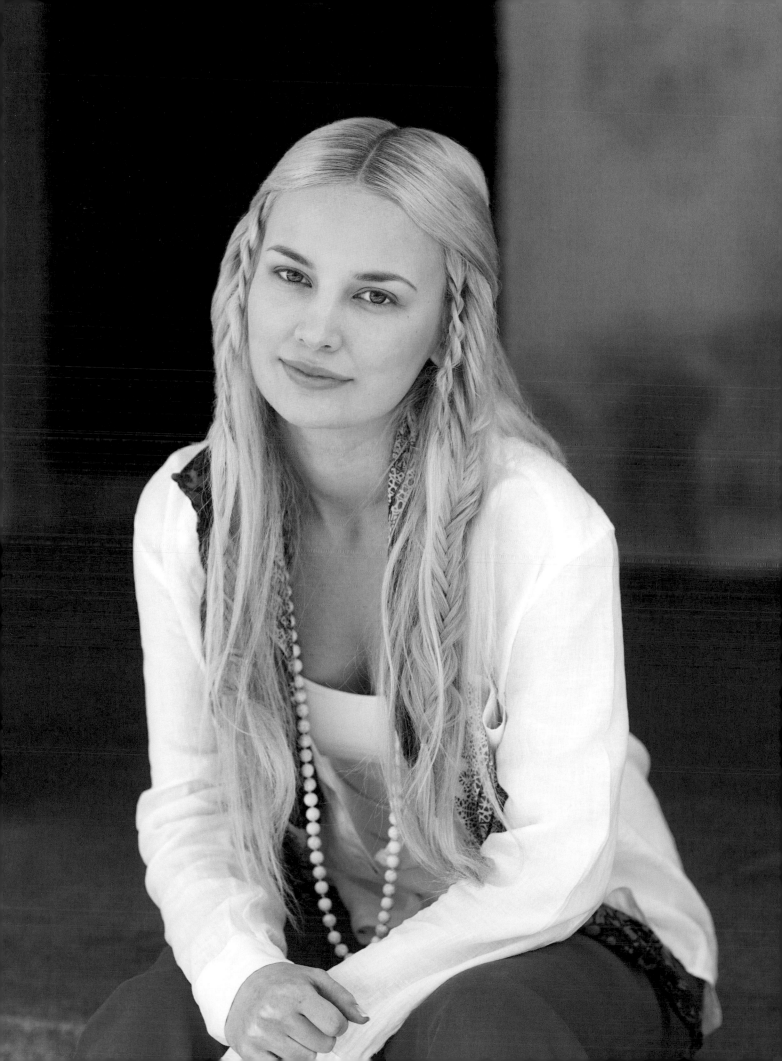

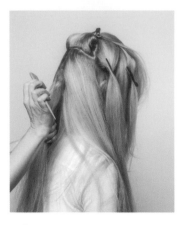

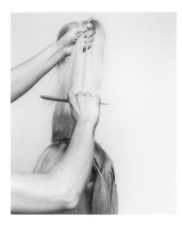

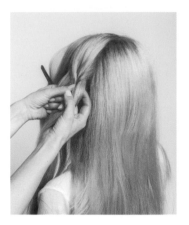

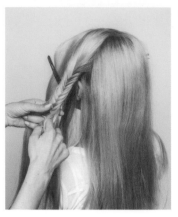

2. Separate a smaller section of hair at the top part of the back of the head. Clip it out of the way with a hair clip.

3. Separate a smaller section from the hair underneath this section and tease part of it with a comb. Unclip the hair from the top section and brush it down toward the neck, to hide the teased hair. This will give you a good foundation for the bang section.

4. Make fishtail braids with the rear side sections by dividing the hair in each section into two parts. Hold one part in each hand. Take a strand from underneath one part and pass it around the section of hair, over the outside edge and across to the opposite side. Switch from one side to the other.

5. Always hold a section of hair in each hand. The thinner the strands you take from each section, the more defined the fishtail pattern will be.

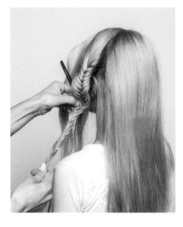

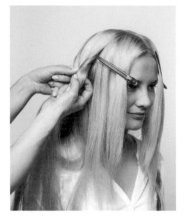

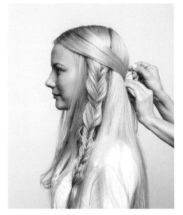

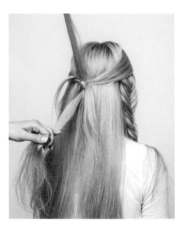

6. Pull at the braid to create more texture. Fasten with an elastic.

7. Repeat steps 4 to 6 for the rear side section on the other side of the head.

8. Take hold of the two front sections. Pull them toward the back of the head and make a knot with the strands. Fasten temporarily with a hairpin.

9. Take up two strands from the loose hair underneath and make two knots on top of the earlier knot. Fasten with a hairpin.

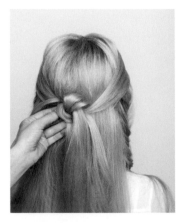

10. Pull at the knot to create a nice shape and fasten with hairpins for stability. Finish with hairspray.

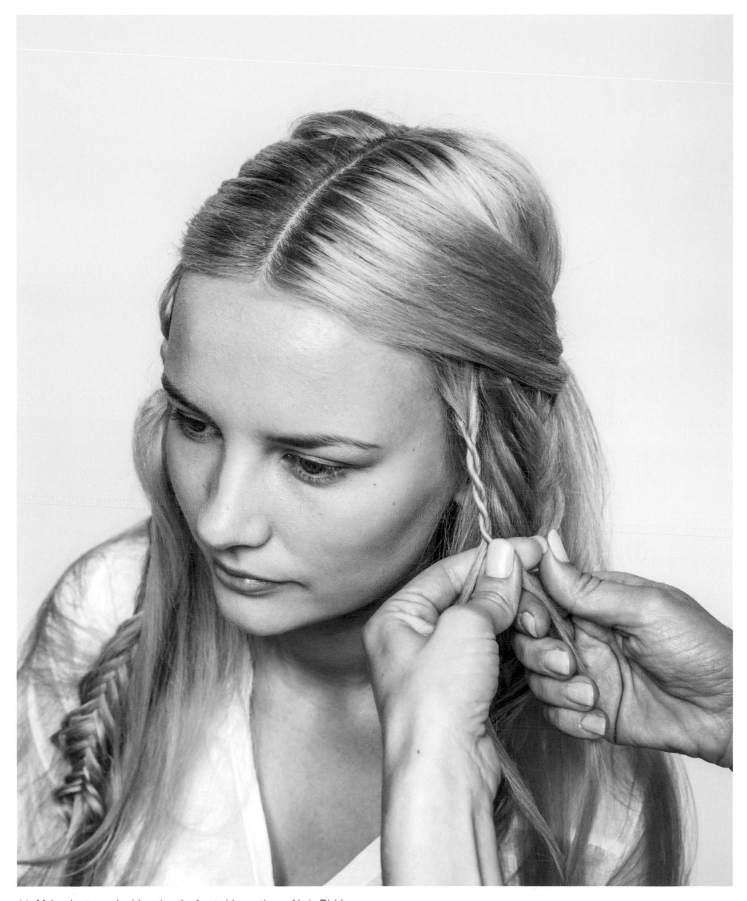

11. Make short rope braids using the front side sections of hair. Divide each section into two parts. Always twist the right strand inward. Switch strands from side to side by twisting the left strand over the right one. Continue twisting. Repeat and work your way down so that a rope-shaped braid takes shape. Tease to set the braids.

Fishtail Bun

Pretty and sophisticated, here four fishtail braids meet in a large bun.

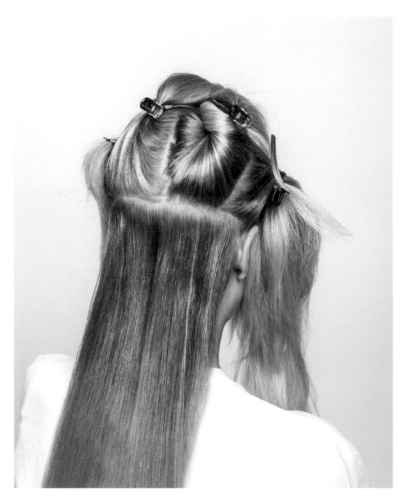

1. Divide the hair into five sections. Draw a part from ear to ear to create a lower section. Then divide the upper hair in four equal-size sections.

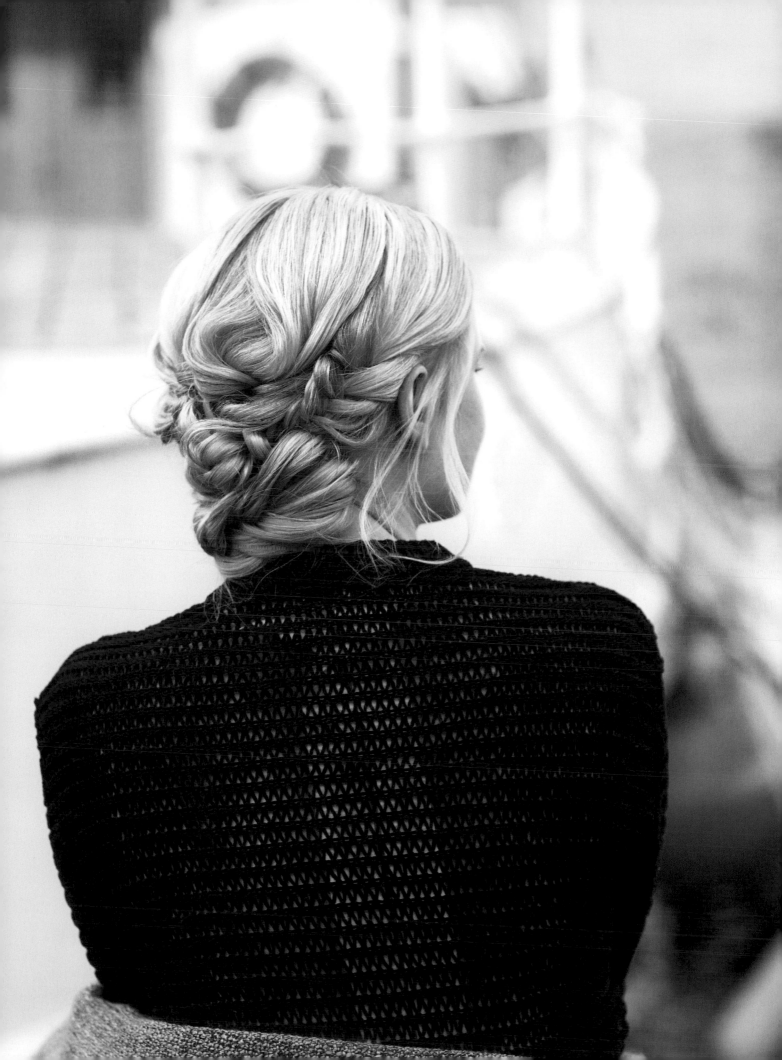

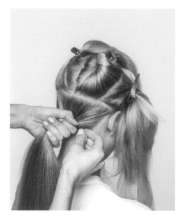

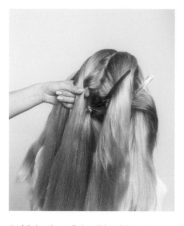

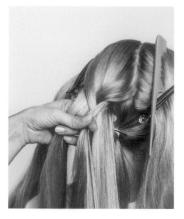

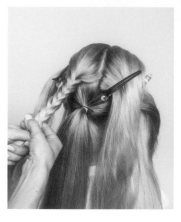

2. Gather the hair in the lower section into a ponytail, low down at the nape of the neck and fasten with an elastic. It's important to make the base of the ponytail stable and steady, since it will be the anchor point for the whole hairstyle.

3. Make four fishtail braids using the upper sections of hair. You may want to use a shine cream as you braid. For each section, divide the hair into two parts. Hold one section of hair in each hand.

4. Take a small strand from the underside of one section. Pass the small strand around the section of hair, over the outside edge and across to the opposite side, and switch from one side to the other.

5. Braid about one-third of the hair length and let the rest of the hair hang free. Fasten with a thin elastic.

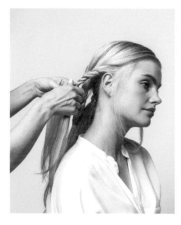

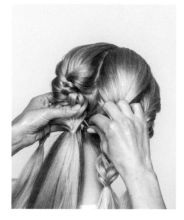

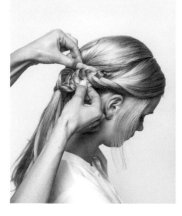

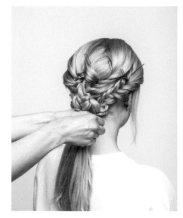

6. Braid the other three sections using the same technique as described in steps 3 to 5.

7. Pull at the braids to add texture. Always pull up from underneath.

8. Lift the braids one by one, pull in toward the center and fasten with hairpins. The unbraided ends of the braids will now meet the lower ponytail.

9. Gather all the hair together and fasten with an elastic.

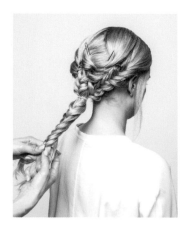

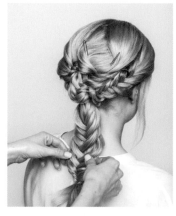

10. Make a fishtail braid from the ponytail, using the technique described in steps 3 to 5.

11. Pull at the braid to give it volume.

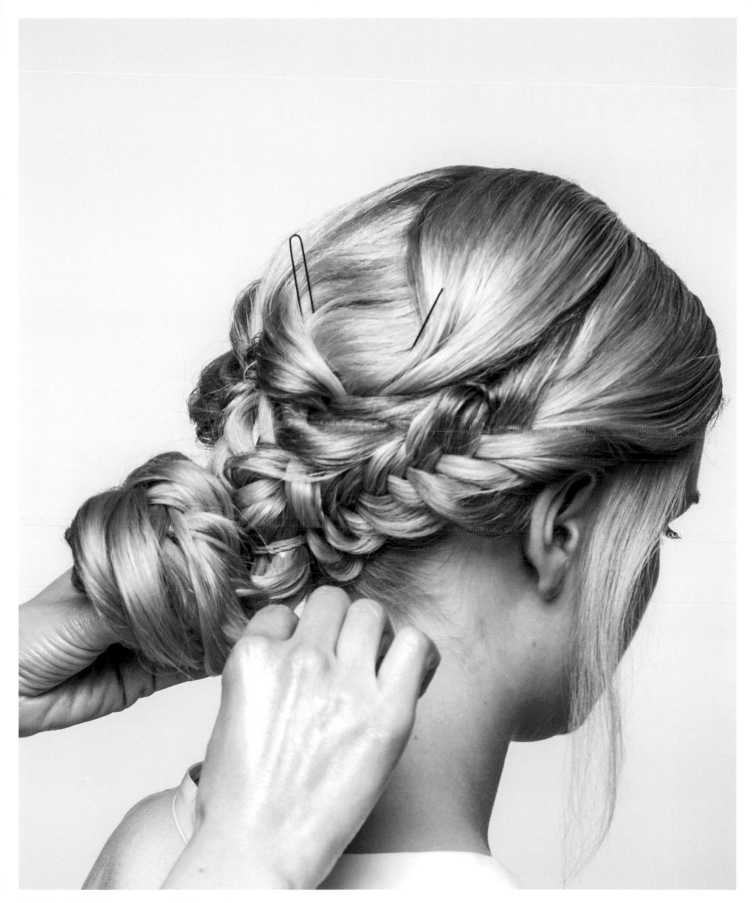

12. Wrap the braid once around the base of the ponytail and fasten with hairpins. Finish with hairspray.

French-braided Fishtail Bun

This fancy updo goes perfectly with an evening gown. The entire head of hair is braided in two fishtail braids that join together— a simple technique with high impact!

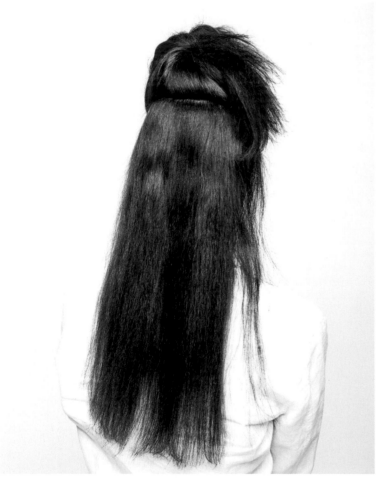

1. Divide the hair into two sections, an upper and a lower section. The part should line up with the end of the eyebrow. Fasten the lower section of hair with a hair clip.

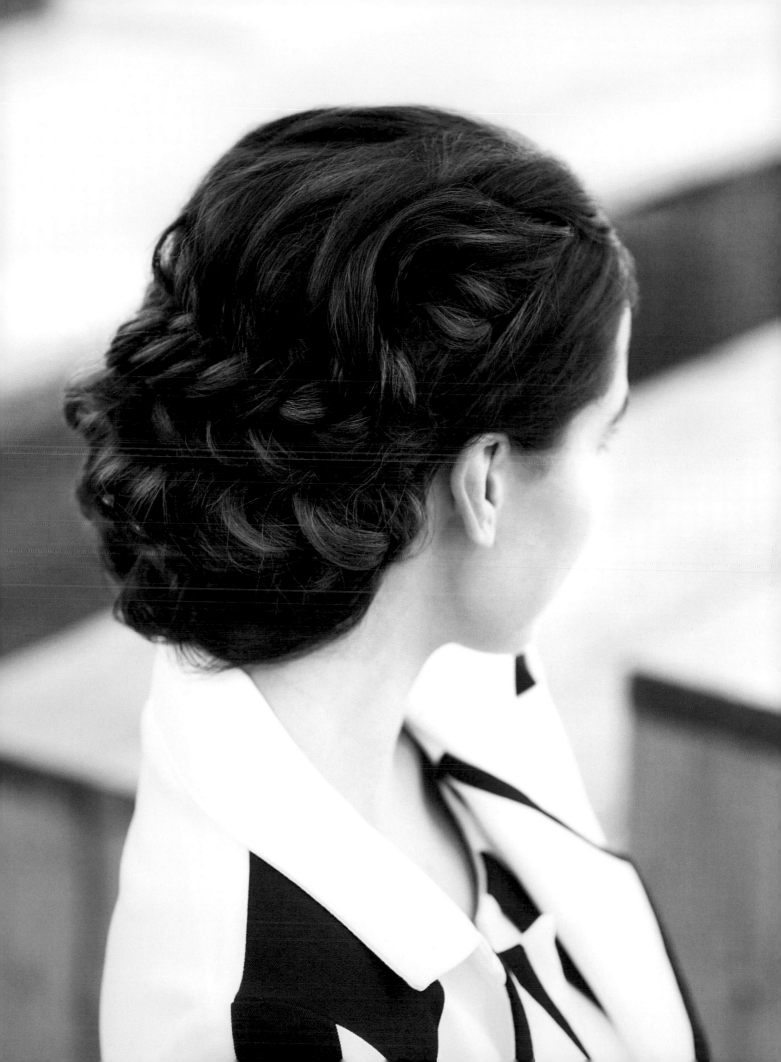

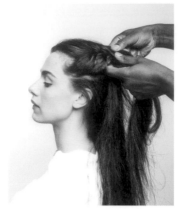

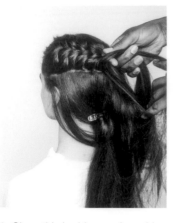

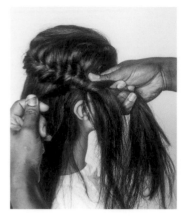

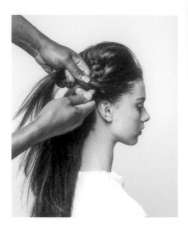

2. Comb through the top section of hair. Make a fishtail braid that runs diagonally across the head down toward the opposite ear. Divide the hair into two parts. Always hold one part in each hand. Take a small strand from underneath one part and pass it around the section of hair at the outside edge and across to the opposite side. Switch from one side to the other.

3. Since this braid runs alongside the head, you will add in new hair as you braid, just as you do with a French braid. The braid will become thinner toward the end and be at its widest at the beginning.

4. When the first braid reaches the other ear, you will unfasten the lower section of hair and begin to integrate it by adding in a strand of hair from the lower section to the first braid.

5. Now twist the braid back and continue to braid downward in the opposite direction by integrating strands from the lower section of hair. Braid using the same technique as in steps 2 and 3. The thinner the strands that you take from each section of hair, the more defined the fishtail pattern will be.

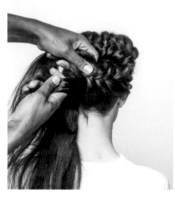

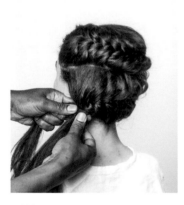

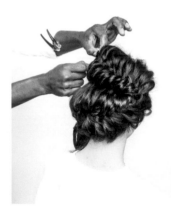

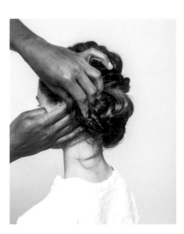

6. The lower braid now runs down toward the shoulder.

7. When the braid reaches the ear-lobe, fasten with an elastic.

8. Begin pulling at the braid in an up and down direction in order to add volume. If you wish, you can pull more at the lower braid to create even more contrast.

9. Take the ends and tuck them in under the braid. Fasten with long hairpins.

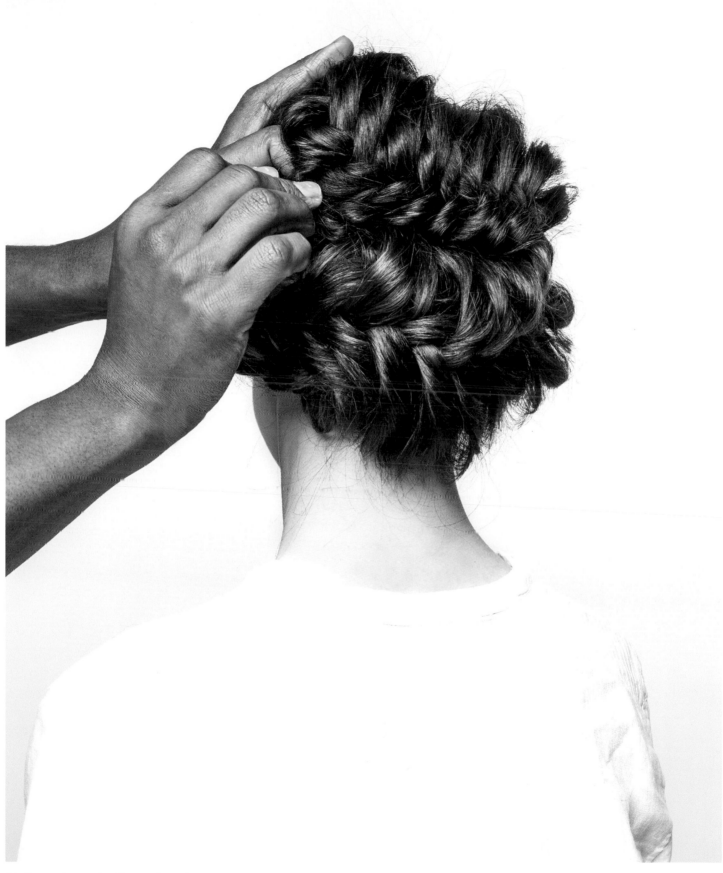

10. Fasten the two braids together using hairpins. Finish with hairspray.

Twin Braid

Create contrast with different-size braids. This hairstyle combines two fishtail braids, one braided tight against the head and the other airy and porous.

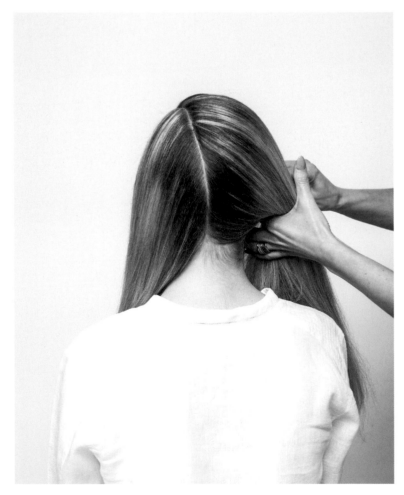

1. Brush through the hair and make a side part.

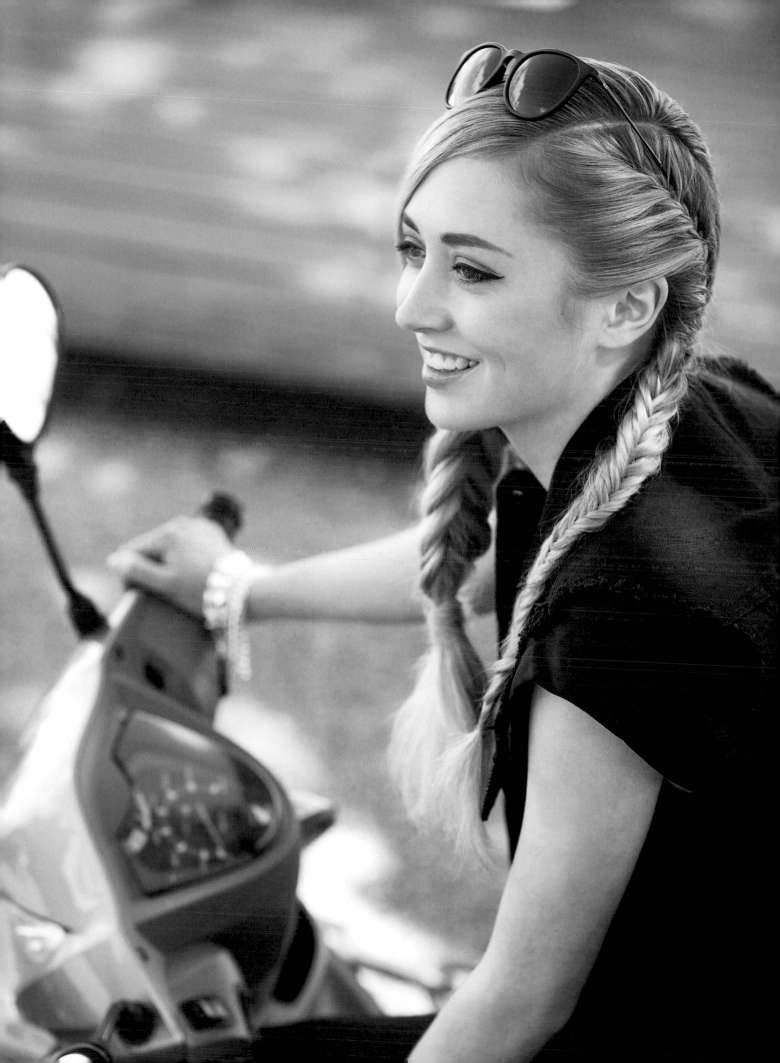

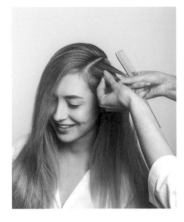

2. Begin with the smaller section of hair. Section out a small piece of hair at the top and near the part, 1.5 inches wide and half an inch thick. Make a French fishtail braid. Divide the hair into two parts. Hold one part in each hand.

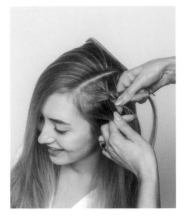

3. Take a small strand from underneath one part and pass it around the section of hair from the outside edge, adding in a new strand from one side and over toward the opposite side. Switch places from one side to the other. Always have a section of hair in each hand.

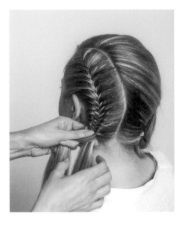

4. Repeat the crossings and add in hair as you braid. Let the braid follow the shape of the head down toward the ear and the shoulder. The thinner the strands that you take from each section, the more defined the fishtail pattern will be.

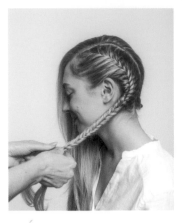

5. Fasten with an elastic.

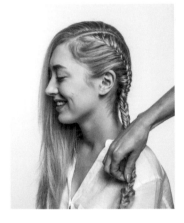

6. Pull at the hair to create more texture, and tease the ends.

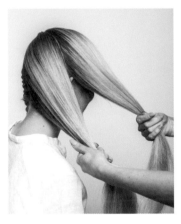

7. Divide the other, larger section of hair into two parts. Hold one part in each hand.

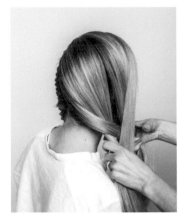

8. Make a fishtail braid. Take a small strand from underneath one part. Pass the small strand around the section of hair from the outside edge and over toward the opposite side. Switch places from one side to the other. Always have a section of hair in each hand.

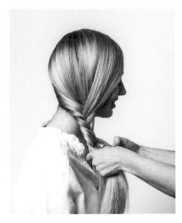

9. Think of braiding in a downward direction, toward the shoulder. Fasten with an elastic.

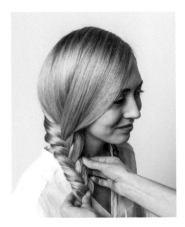

10. Pull at the braid to create more volume.

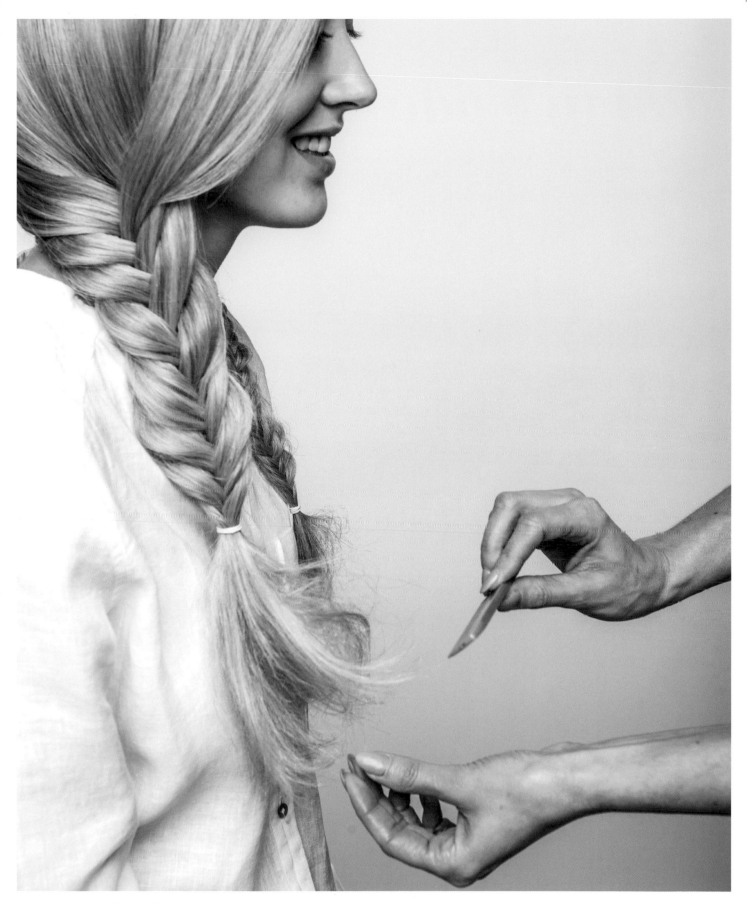

11. Tease the ends. Finish with hairspray.

Party Updo

A classic hairstyle with 1960s vibes, the knotted French braids give plenty of texture to the updo.

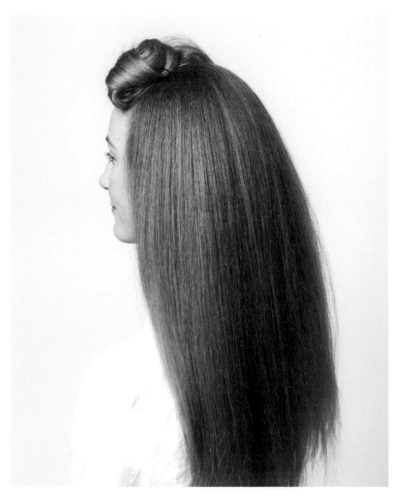

1. Separate the bang section and clip out of the way with a hair clip.

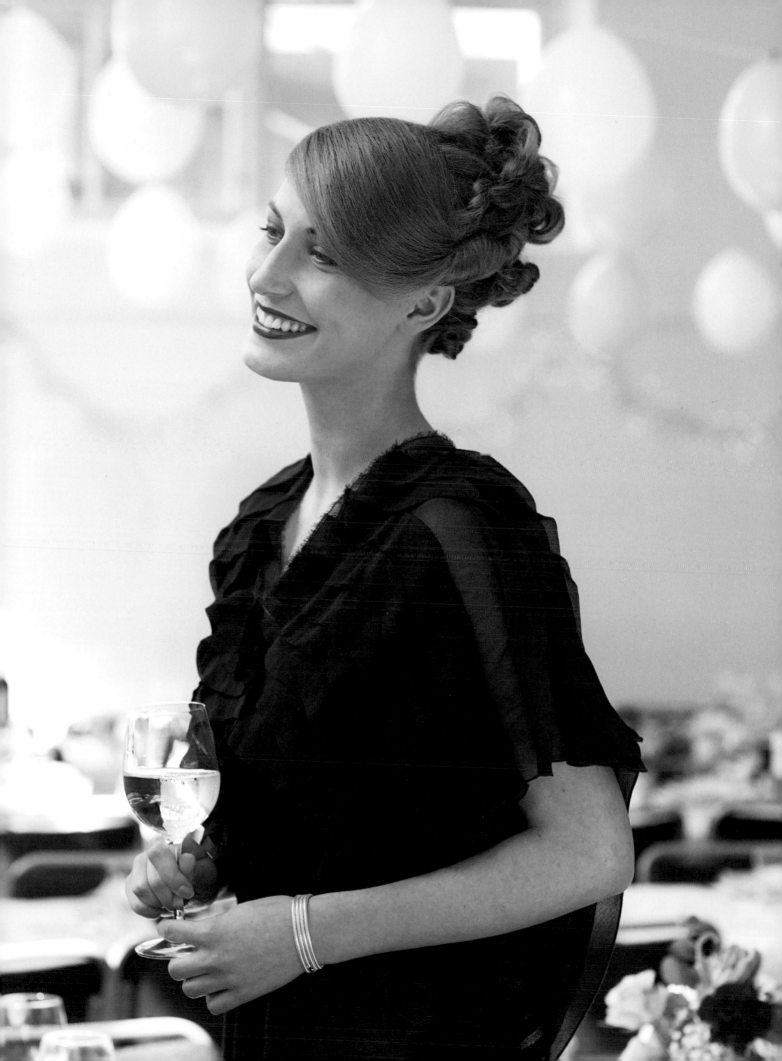

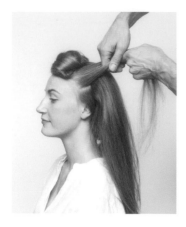

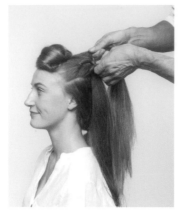

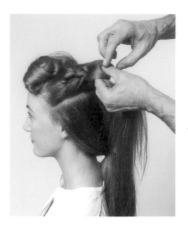

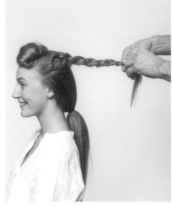

2. Create a section on one side of the face by drawing a part 1 inch above the ear. The section should make up one-third of the hair. Temporarily fasten the remaining lower section of hair with an elastic.

3. Now you will make a knotted French braid using the side section. Pick up a small piece of hair from the front part of the section. Divide into two strands. Make a knot.

4. Continue knotting the strands as you add in more hair, just as when you make a French braid.

5. Repeat the knotting until the entire length is used up. Fasten with an elastic. Temporarily pin the braid on top of the head.

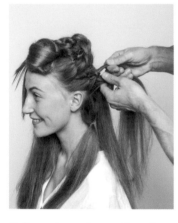

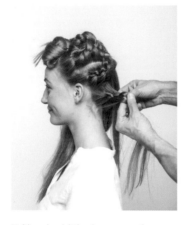

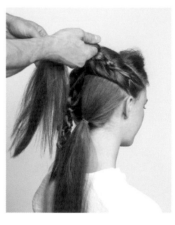

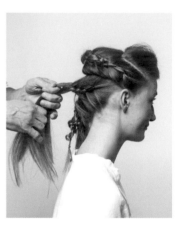

6. Separate another section of the lower hair. This section should make up half of the hair. Repeat the technique described in steps 3 to 5.

7. Now braid the lower section in the same way as described in steps 3 to 5.

8. Braid the opposite side. Divide the hair into two equal sections, upper and lower. Fasten the lower section temporarily with an elastic. Follow steps 3 to 5. Braid diagonally upward to achieve the right effect. Fasten with an elastic.

9. Now braid the lower section of hair in the same way as in steps 3 to 5. Point the braid in toward the center of the head.

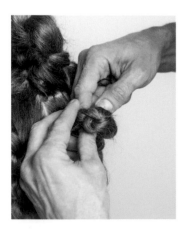

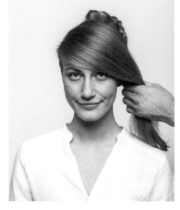

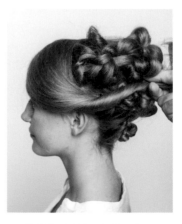

10. Fold in the ends and fasten with hairpins.

11. Let down the bang section. As a contrast to the braid, the bangs should be sleek and sweep alongside the face before being attached to the bun.

12. Pull the hair back. Starting at the ear, twist the hair and fasten to the braid using hairpins.

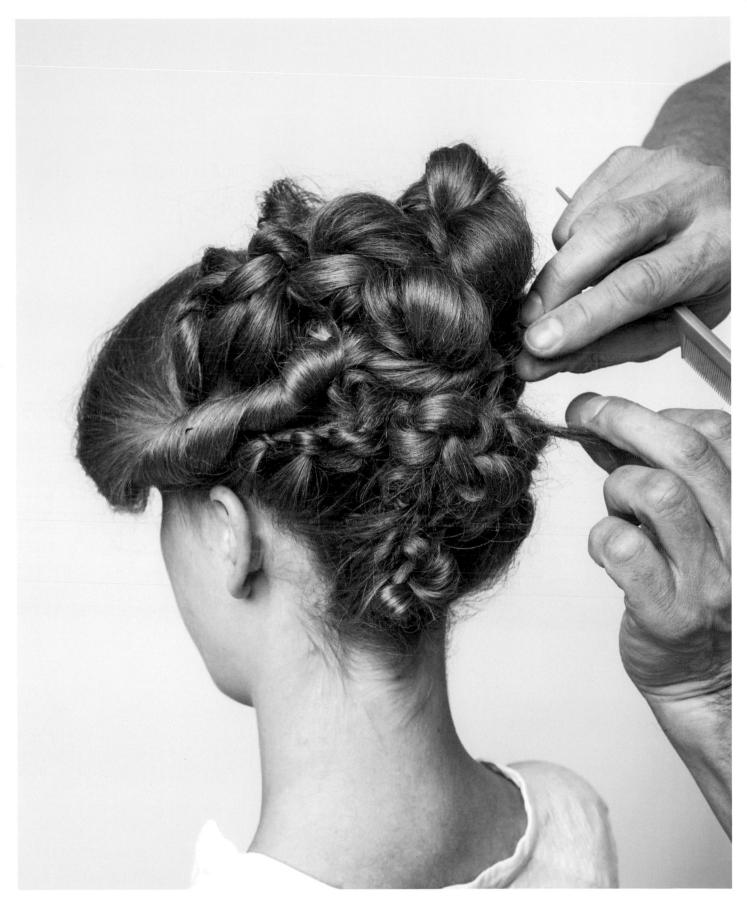

13. Pull at the braids to create more volume and texture in the style. Set with hairspray.

Retro Bun

By crimping the hair before braiding, you can give your braids lots of volume and high impact. Here we use simple knotted braids to create a unique hairstyle.

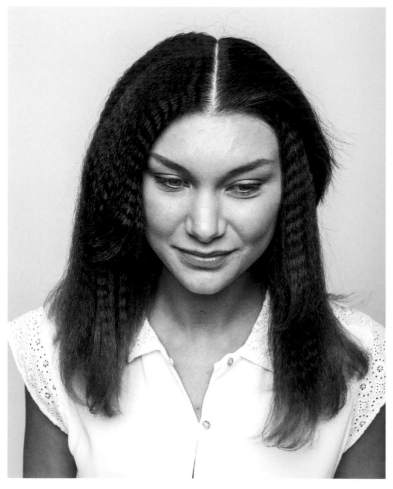

1. Prepare the hair by using a crimping iron. The hair will be lightly waved throughout its length. Divide the hair with a center part.

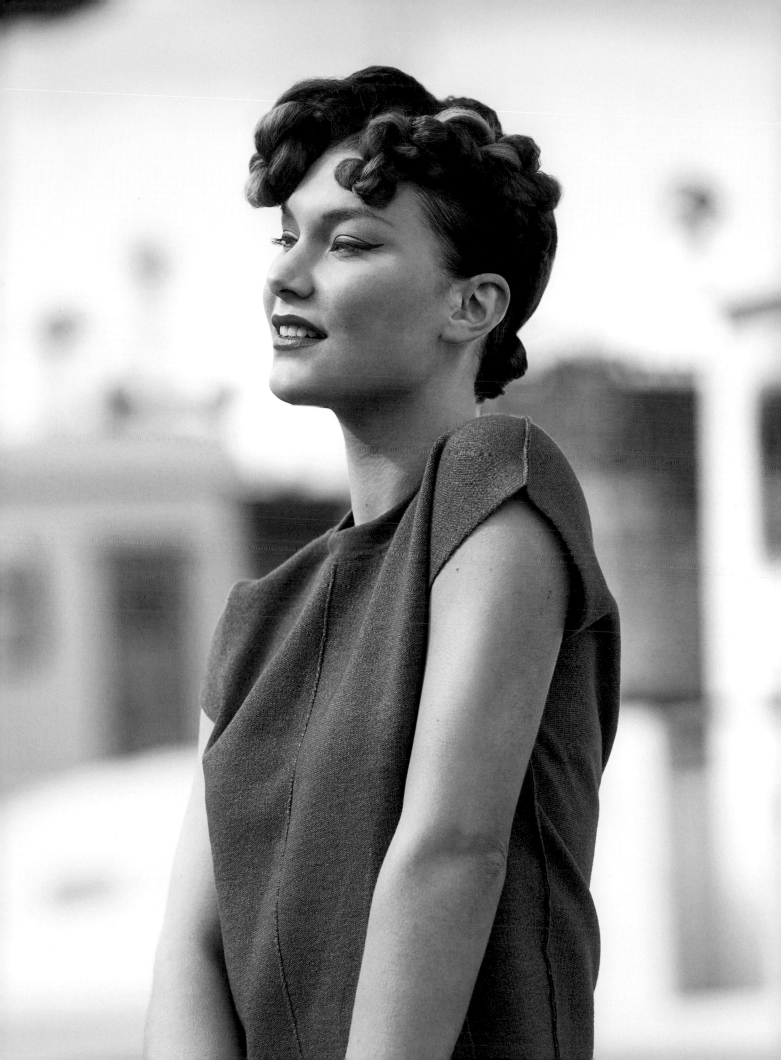

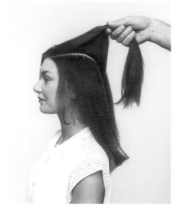

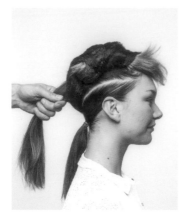

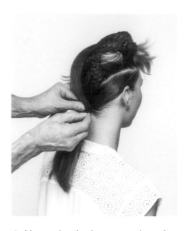

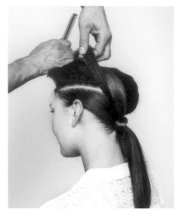

2. Draw another part to the right of the center part. This part is also straight but runs diagonally from the forehead for an asymmetrical feel. This section of hair should be about 2 inches wide. Fasten with a clip.

3. Gather the lower section of hair into a ponytail low down at the nape of the neck.

4. Now take the loose section of hair on the side, by the ear, and twist it around the base of the ponytail. Fasten with short hairpins.

5. Next you will make a knotted braid using the section closest to the center part. Begin at the neck and braid upward toward the crown. Section out a piece of hair at the neck and divide into two strands.

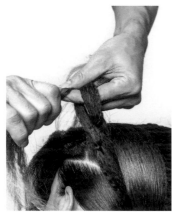

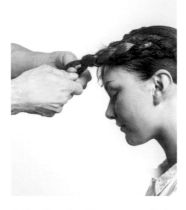

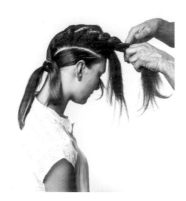

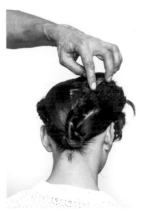

6. Make a knot with the strands, section out another piece of hair and tie another knot.

7. Continue knotting as you add in hair. Fasten with a small elastic.

8. Now continue with the other section. Braid in the same way as in steps 5 and 6. Begin at the neck, moving up toward the face.

9. When you are done with the braids, twist the ponytail at the neck and turn it upward. Lock in place with a pair of hairpins.

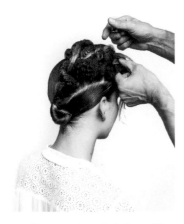

10. Use extra large hairpins to lift the braids and give the hairstyle some height. Fasten with hairpins.

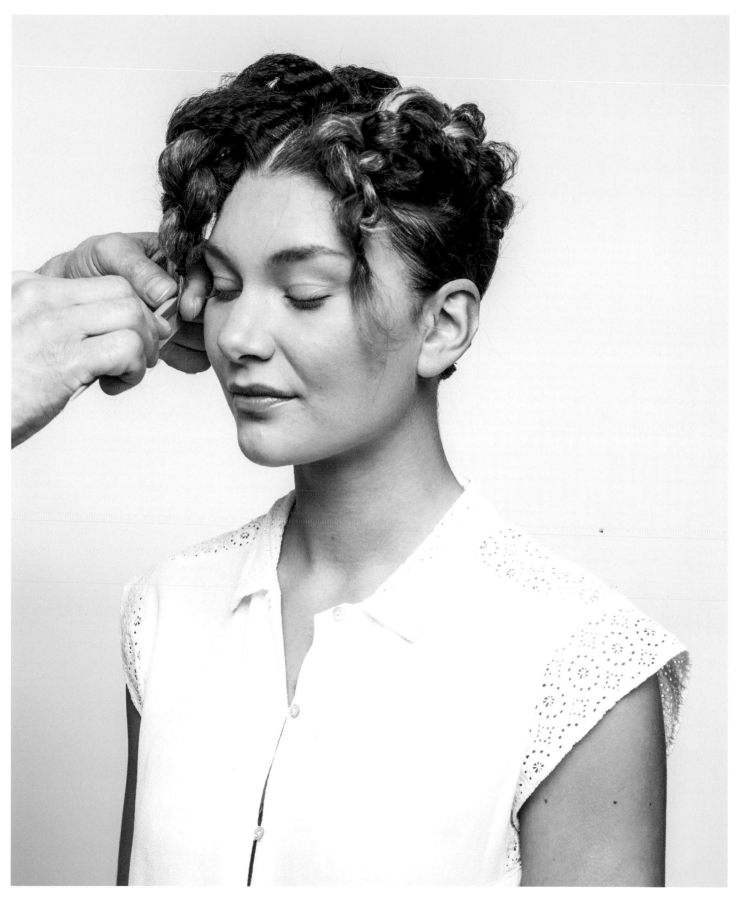

11. Pull at the braid to create the feeling you
want. Tease the ends. Finish with hairspray.

Grace Kelly

An updo that exudes elegance, this hairstyle might look advanced, but it's easy to create. Loose knotted braids create a pretty design and high volume.

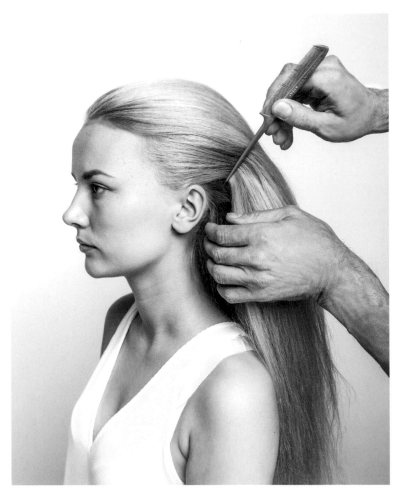

1. Brush the hair back. Use hairspray to brush in stray ends.

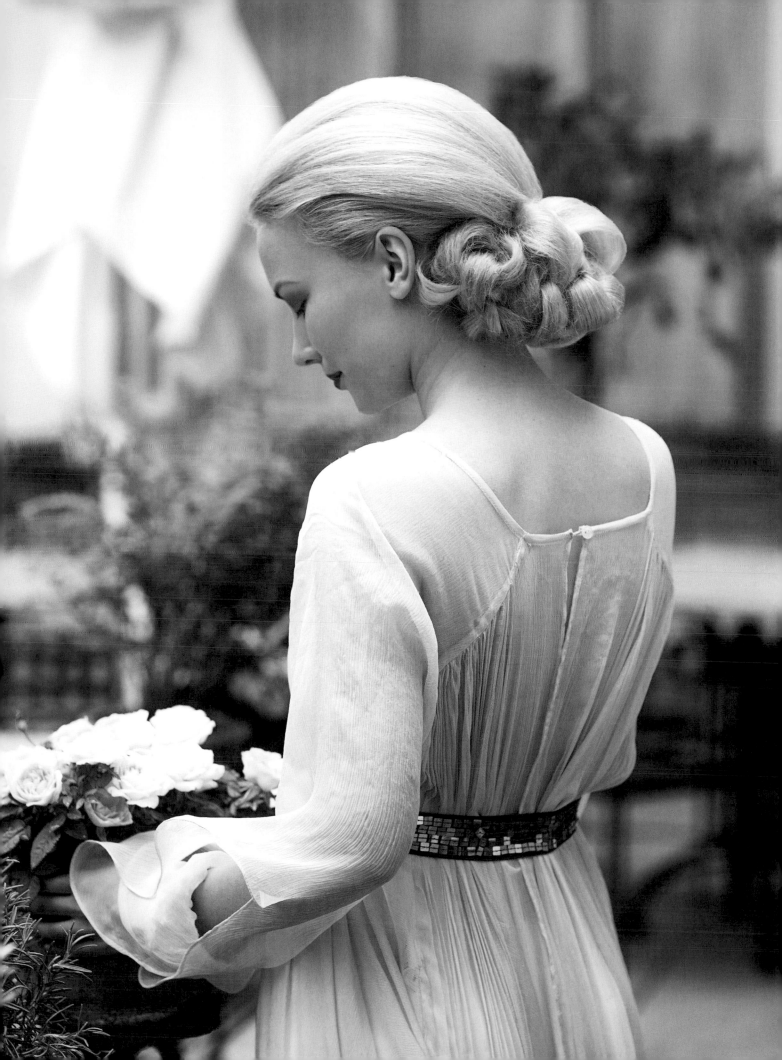

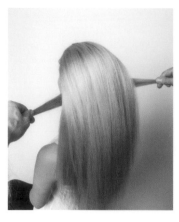

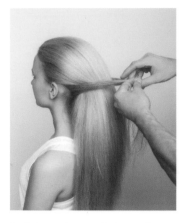

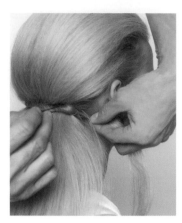

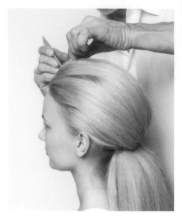

2. Separate two small sections of hair behind each ear, about 1 inch wide. Hold one section in each hand.

3. Twist each strand, then twist the two strands together and pull the ends.

4. Fasten the twisted strands with hairpins.

5. Using a rattail comb, lift the upper hair to create volume.

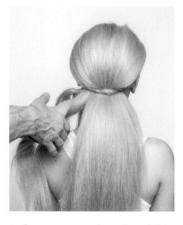

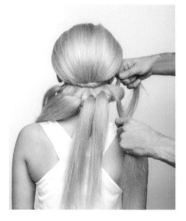

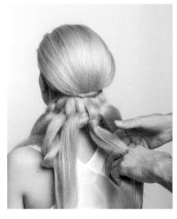

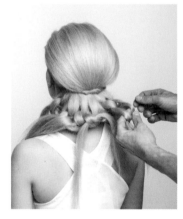

6. Separate a small section, divide into two strands and make a loose knot.

7. Repeat until you have worked through the entire section.

8. Repeat knotting, using two strands at a time. Work from one side to the other.

9. Repeat step 6 until the entire hair is knotted.

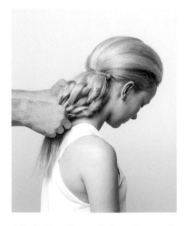

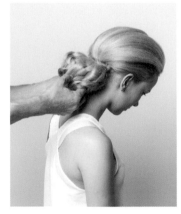

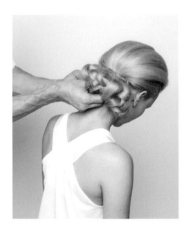

10. Gather the ends together and fasten with an elastic.

11. Fold the ends toward the anchored hair at the neck.

12. Fasten with hairpins.

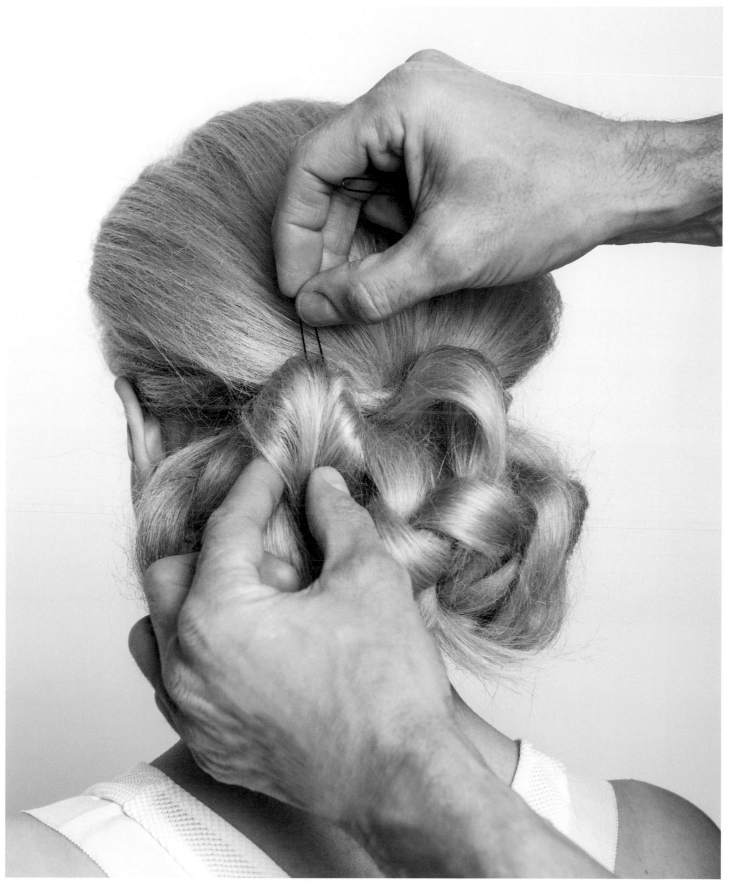

13. Now you can begin to experiment with the style. Pull at the bun to create more volume, and fasten with small hairpins. Finish with hairspray.

Paris Bun

This hairstyle combines an updo with loose hair. Four different knotted braids create a striking shape on top of the head.

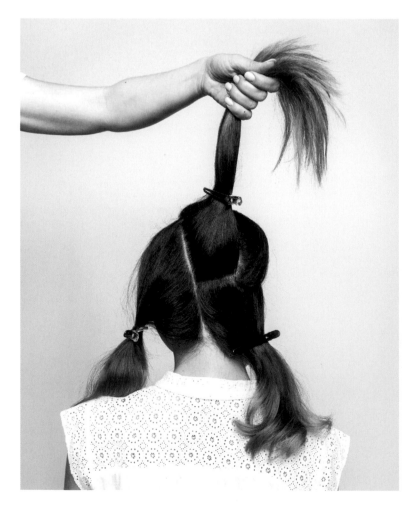

1. Divide the hair into four sections. Draw a part on the left side, up toward the crown and then down to the center of the neck. Draw a part beginning from the same place as the previous part, and pull the part straight back in the center but stop where the back of the head begins to curve. You will be left with a wedge about 1 inch wide from the forehead down to the curve of the head between the two parts. Make a third part on the right side of the face, level with the midpoint of the eyebrow, which turns diagonally downward toward the opposite ear.

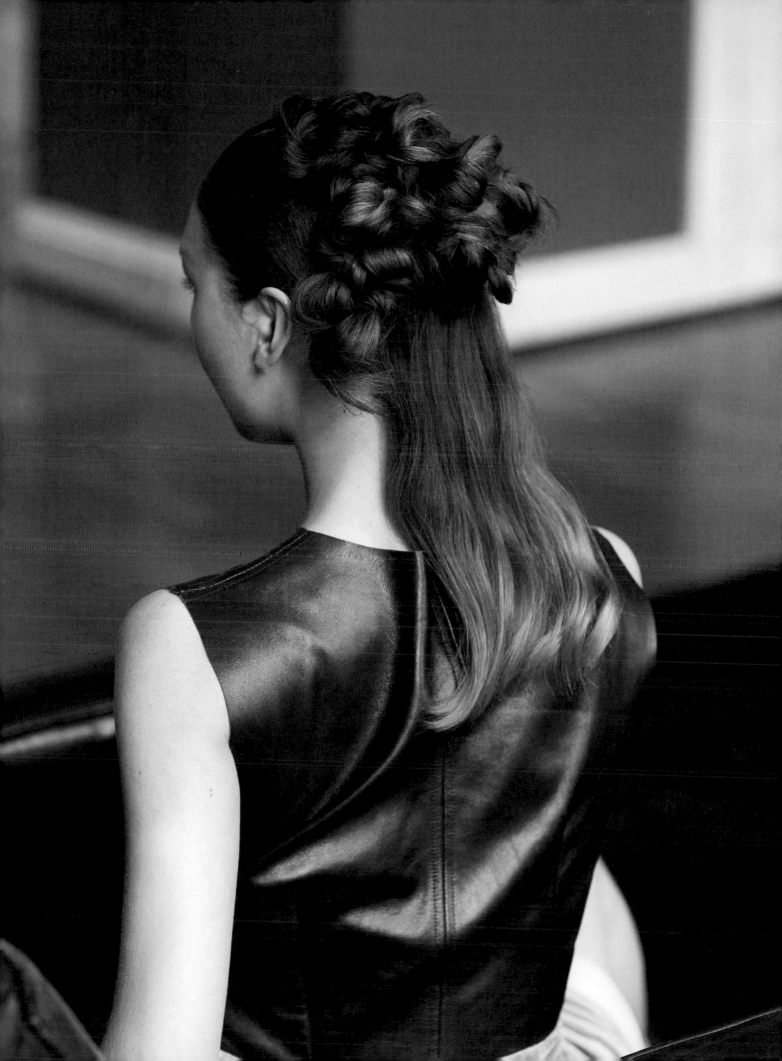

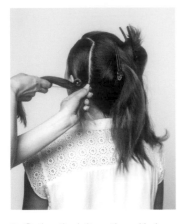

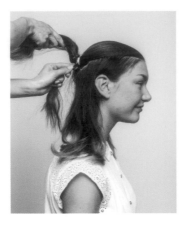

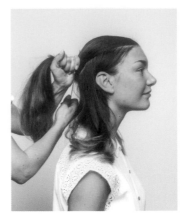

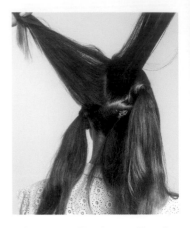

2. Gather the left section of hair and make a ponytail behind the ear and low down near the neck. Fasten with an elastic.

3. Section out a strand from the ponytail and twist it. Wrap the strand around the base of the ponytail to hide the elastic. Fasten with a small hairpin. Clip the pony-tail out of the way.

4. Gather the upper right section of hair into a ponytail placed at the back where the head curves, and fasten with an elastic. Conceal the elastic in the same way as in step 3.

5. Now you will make two French-knotted braids using the section of hair between the two ponytails. Divide this section into two smaller parts.

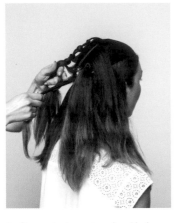

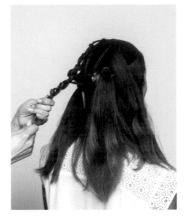

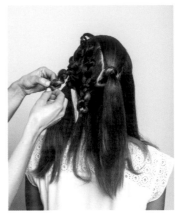

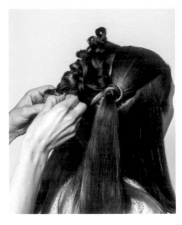

6. Separate two strands of hair from one section. Make a loose knot with the strands. Take hold of the strands and repeat to make a new knot. Think of making loose knots with a large loops. Continue to add in hair from the as you knot.

7. Leave about 4 inches of the length unbraided. Fasten with an elastic. Repeat the same tech-nique as described in step 6 to braid the other section of hair.

8. Pull at the braids to create more texture. Work from the bottom up.

9. Lift the braid onto the head and fasten with a hairpin. Continue pull-ing at the braid until you have a shape that you like.

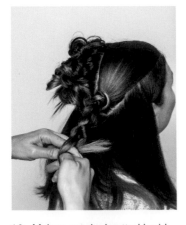

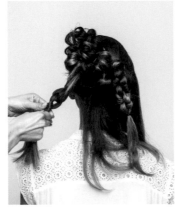

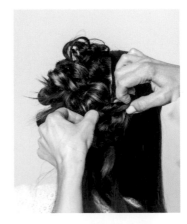

10 . Make a regular knotted braid with each of the two ponytails. Divide one ponytail into two smaller sections. Make a loose knot with the strands. Repeat to make a new knot. Fasten with an elastic.

11. Repeat step 10 and make a knotted braid with the other pony-tail. Fasten this one as well with an elastic.

12. Pull at the braids to create more texture. Begin at the bottom and work your way up.

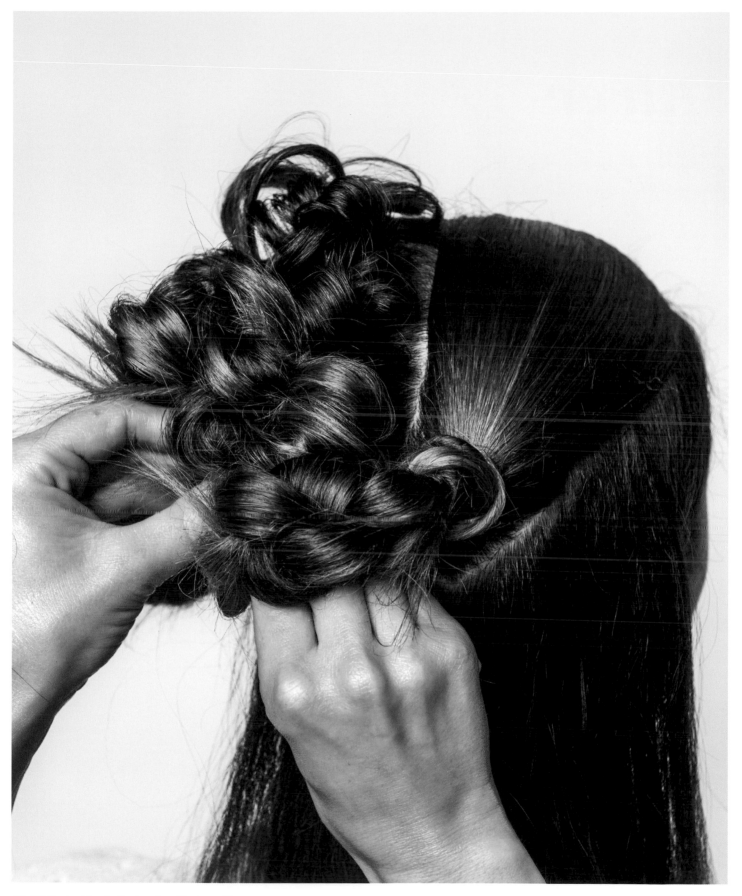

13. Lift the braid onto the head and fasten with
a hairpin. Continue pulling at the braid until you
have a shape that you like. Let the lower hair
hang free. Comb through the loose hair. Finish
with hairspray.

River

Sweep all the hair back into an elegant knotted braid. This hairstyle is easy to make and works for any occasion!

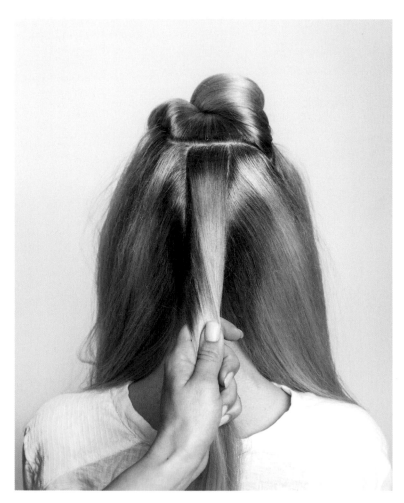

1. Brush the hair back. Separate the hair at the crown of the head and fasten with a clip. Divide the rest of the hair into three sections, two large sections on each side of the face and one smaller section, about 1 inch wide, in the center.

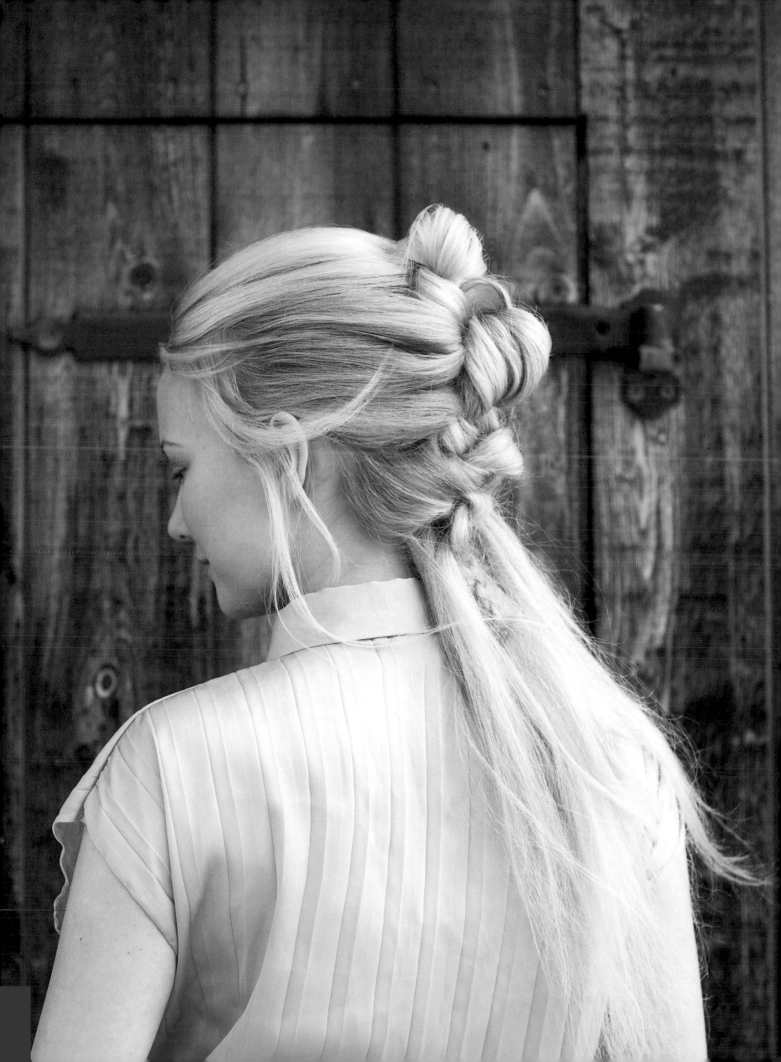

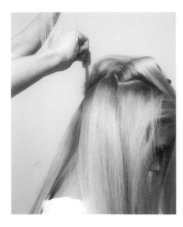

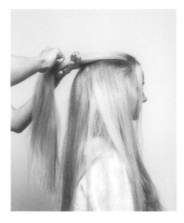

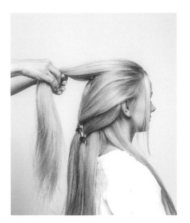

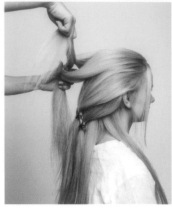

2. Tease the midsection to create an anchor point.

3. Separate out two smaller pieces of hair on each side of the face, about 1 to 1.25 inches wide. Fasten together with a hair clip.

4. Repeat step 3 with the other section.

5. Remove the clip from the crown hair and brush through with fingers. Divide into two smaller sections and make a knot. Fasten with a hairpin.

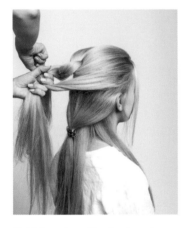

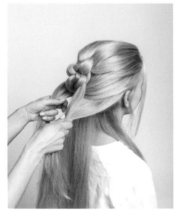

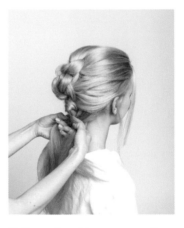

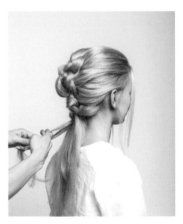

6. Make yet another knot, and fasten with a hairpin.

7. Now continue working your way down by tying the smaller sections that you separated out in steps 3 and 4. Make sure you pull the hair backward and upward as you knot. Fasten each knot with a hairpin.

8. Separate out two more sections in the remaining hair. Tie a knot and fasten with a hairpin.

9. Catch up two smaller strands and tie a smaller knot to finish the braid.

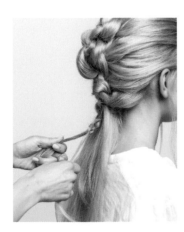

10. Now pick up two smaller strands and tie these to the ends, as a finishing detail for the hairstyle.

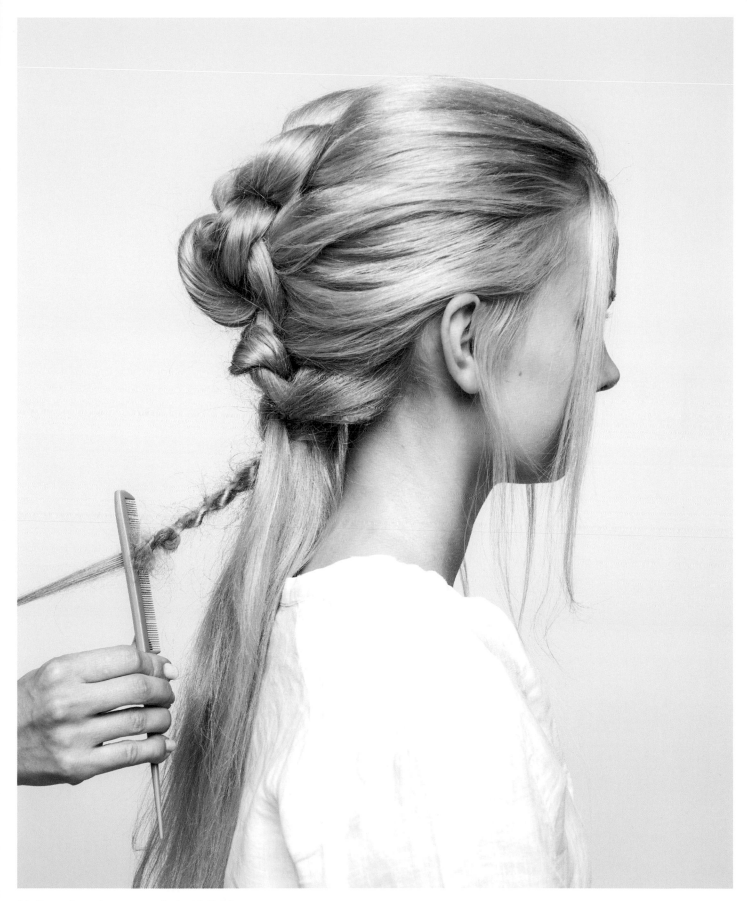

11. Tease the ends to secure the braid. Finish
with hairspray.

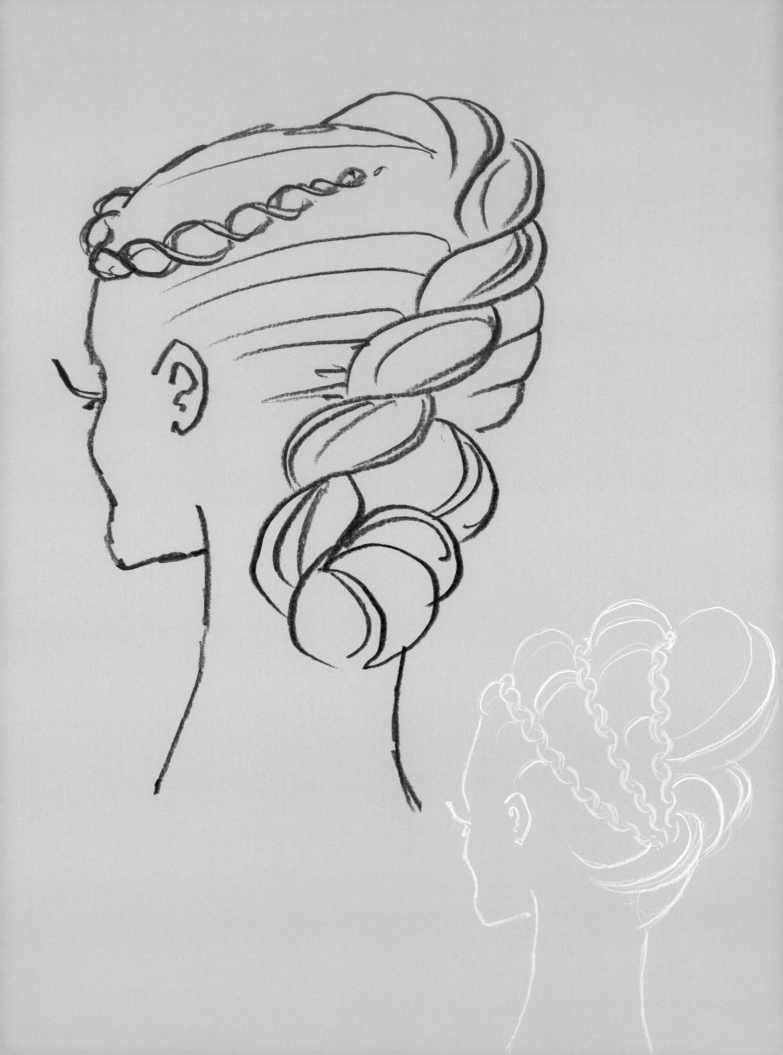

Rope
Braids

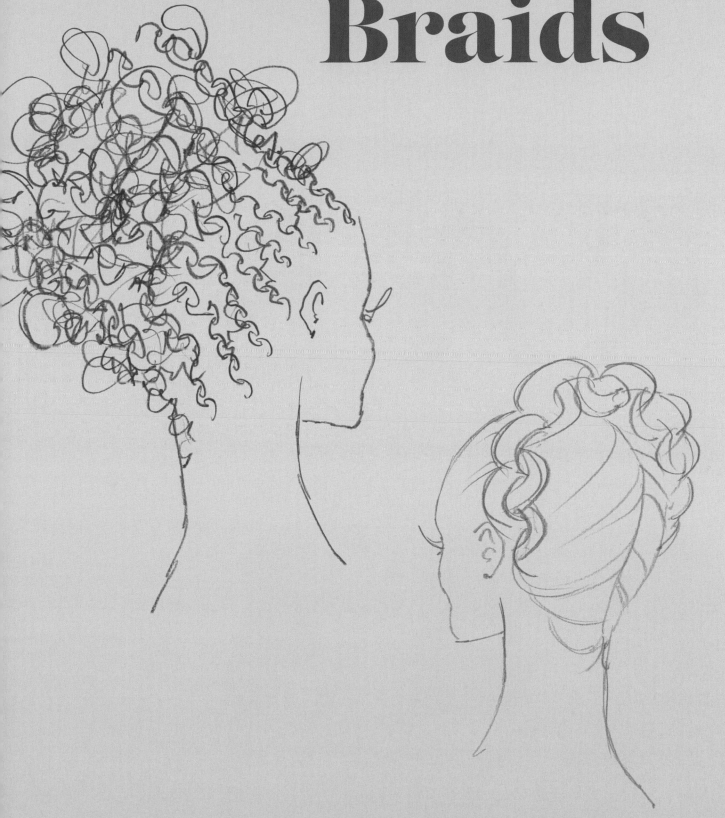

Twisted Waterfall Braid

This is a practical everyday style that is suitable for most hair lengths and is beautiful in its simplicity!

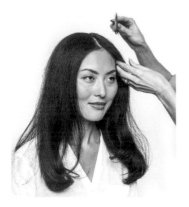

1. Divide the hair into two sections by making a straight center part.

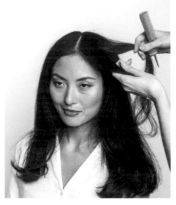

2. Separate out a smaller section in the upper part of the hair at one side, slightly more than 1 inch wide. Divide this section into two strands.

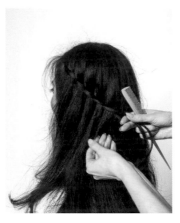

3. Now you will make a rope braid. Wrap the strands around each other. Begin twisting with the lower strand. When you have made one round, pick up a strand from the upper part of the hair and pass it through the twist.

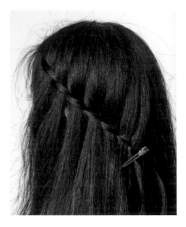

4. Repeat step 3 as you work down toward the neck. Between rounds you can comb the underneath hair to keep it smooth and neat. When you come to the end of the braid, fasten temporarily with a hair clip.

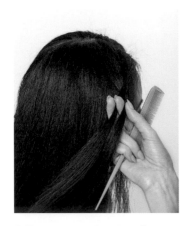

5. Repeat steps 2 to 4 on the other side of the hair. Twist down toward the neck. The braids should meet in a V-shape at the neck.

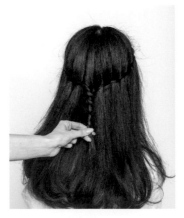

6. Bring the braids together and twist them down toward the back. Fasten with an elastic.

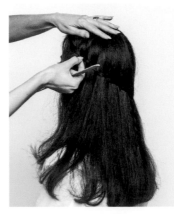

7. Lighten up the braids in front by pulling carefully at them. Finish with a shine spray.

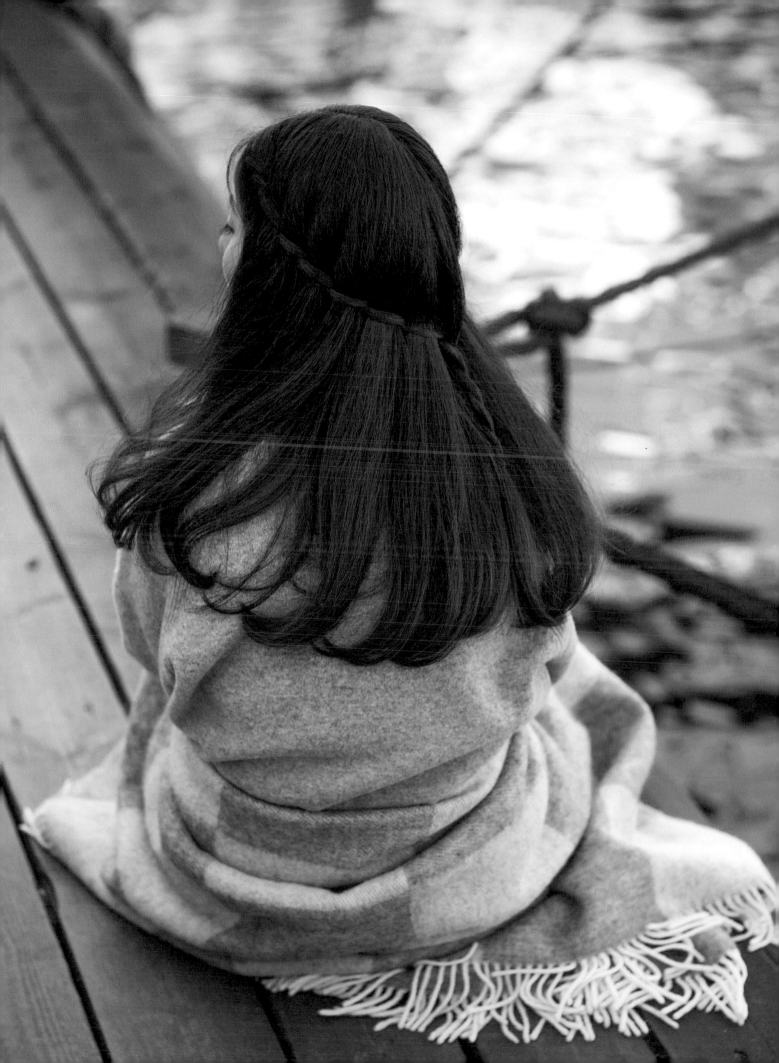

Asymmetrical Rope Braid

This is a sophisticated hairstyle where two French rope braids are gathered into an updo on one side of the head. Simple and striking!

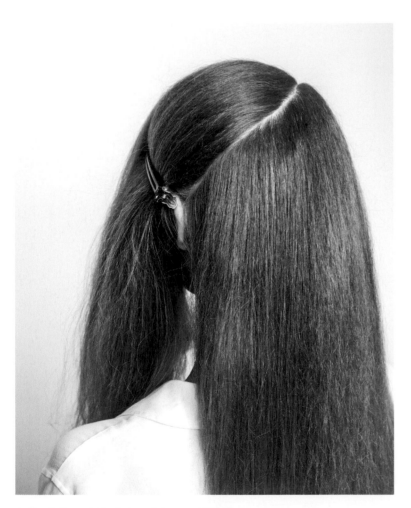

1. Brush through the hair and draw a side part, beginning from a point lined up with the center of one eyebrow and going down toward the opposite ear.

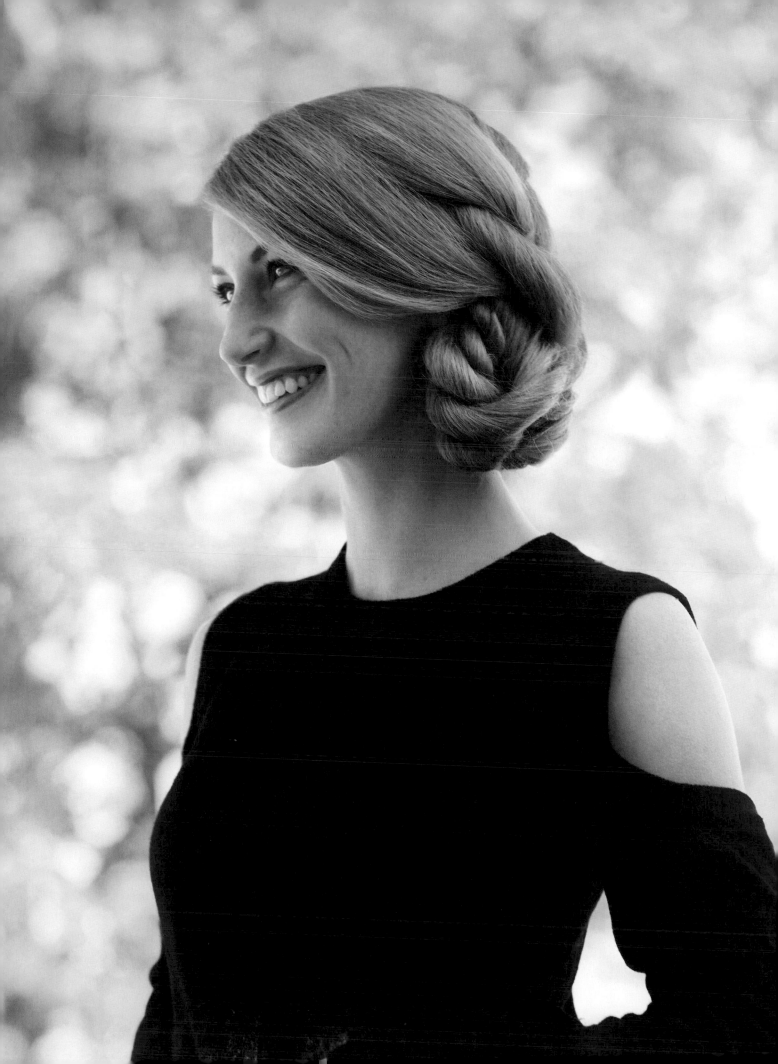

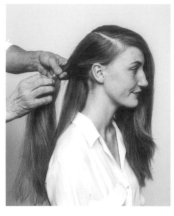

2. Make a French rope braid with the lower section of hair. Divide this section into two strands on the right side. Always twist the right-most strand inward. Switch sides by crossing the left strand over the right one. At the same time you will add in more hair from the part that is hanging free. Switch sides again and repeat until a rope-shaped braid takes shape.

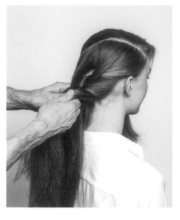

3. Add in new hair for each round. Braid alongside the head in a diagonal downward direction.

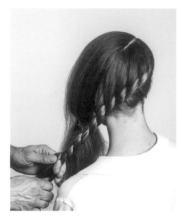

4. Braid the entire length and fasten with an elastic.

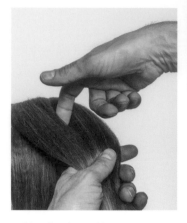

5. Now begin working on the front section of hair. Section out a part of the bangs.

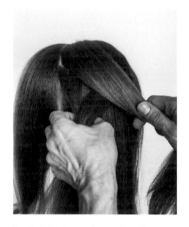

6. Braid this section using the same technique as described in step 2.

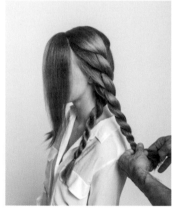

7. The French rope braid should point down toward the shoulder. Braid the entire length.

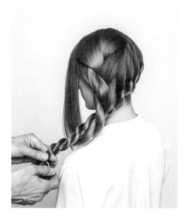

8. Twist the two braids together. Fasten with an elastic.

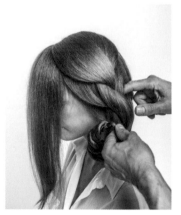

9. Pull the ends of the braid up through the upper part of the braid.

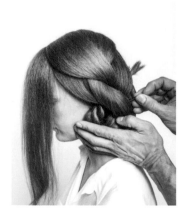

10. Secure with hairpins. Set with hairspray.

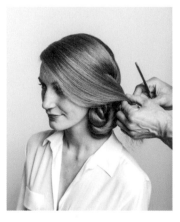

11. Now sweep the bang section down toward the braid.

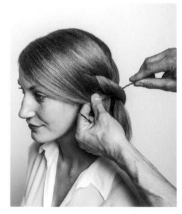

12. Attach the bang section to the braid using two extra long hairpins. Slide one pin into the bang section and pull through the hair using the other pin.

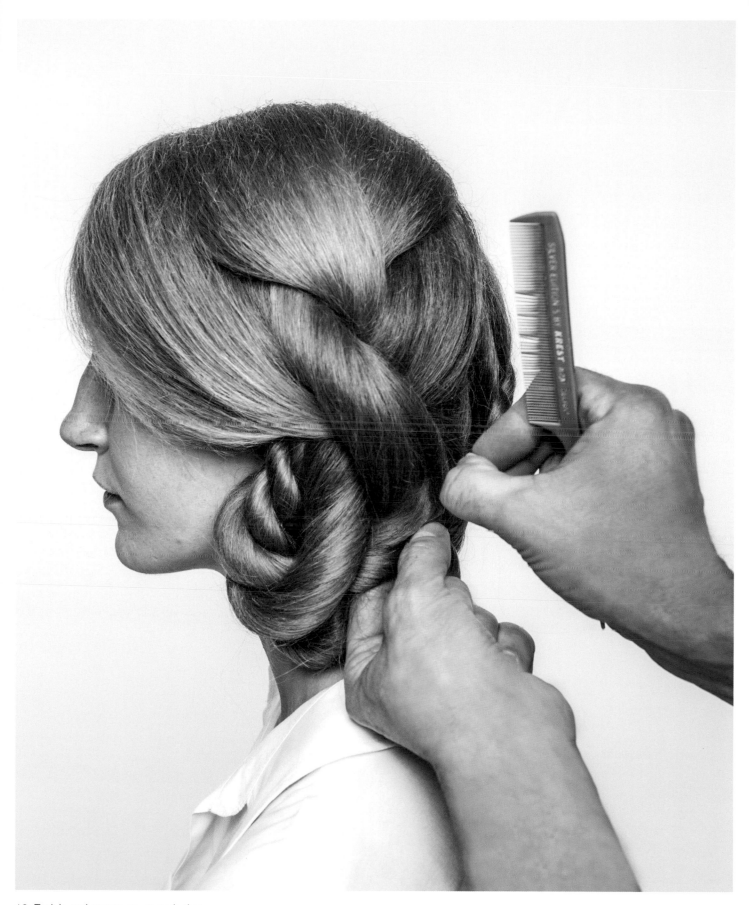

13. Tuck in and secure any strands that may
stick out from the hairstyle. Finish with hairspray.

Deluxe Rope Braid

This hairstyle looks advanced but is actually simple to make. It consists of three airy French rope braids that can easily be expanded for a fuller look, and you can shape it any way you like. Don't be afraid to experiment with both height and volume!

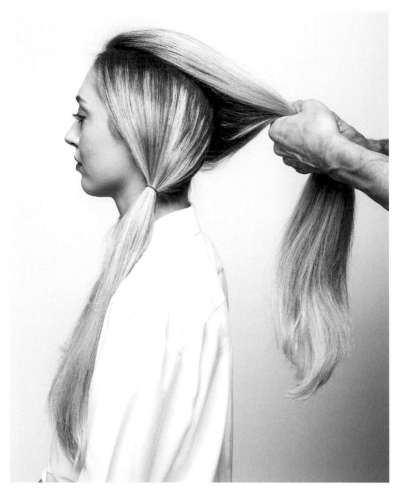

1. Divide the hair into three sections by creating a V-shaped part from the center of the forehead. Fasten the two side sections with elastics.

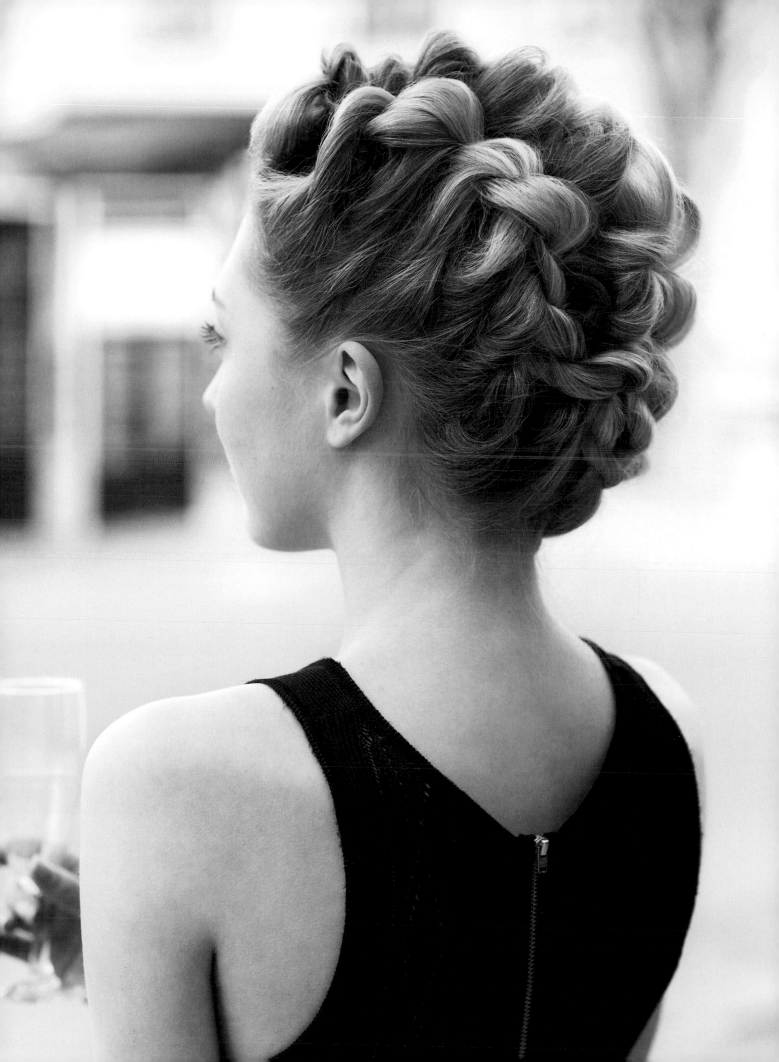

134

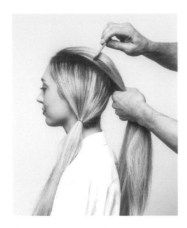

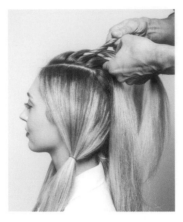

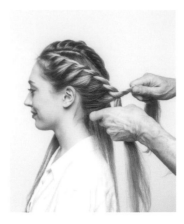

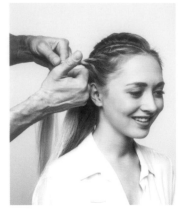

2. Begin with the midsection. Divide this section into two strands.

3. Twist the right strand inward. Switch the two strands by crossing the left over the right, while adding in new hair from the part that is hanging free. Twist the new strand, on the right, inward. Change places again, adding in new hair for each round. Twist loosely. Braid the entire length of hair. Fasten with an elastic.

4. Now continue with one of the side sections. Separate out a section at the front and divide into two strands. Repeat the technique described in step 3, but this time only add in hair from the outside edge. Twist the braid inward, toward the neck.

5. Repeat step 3 for the other side section.

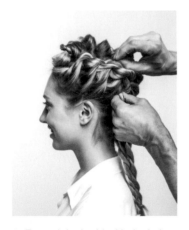

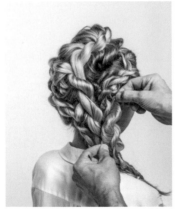

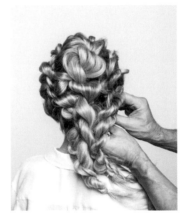

6. Expand the braid with the help of long hairpins. Lift the braid with one hand as you insert a long hairpin with the other hand. Each braid must be lifted and fastened with two or three hairpins.

7. Pull at the braids with your fingers, as much as you can without making them disintegrate.

8. Create an anchor point under the braids using a few bobby pins.

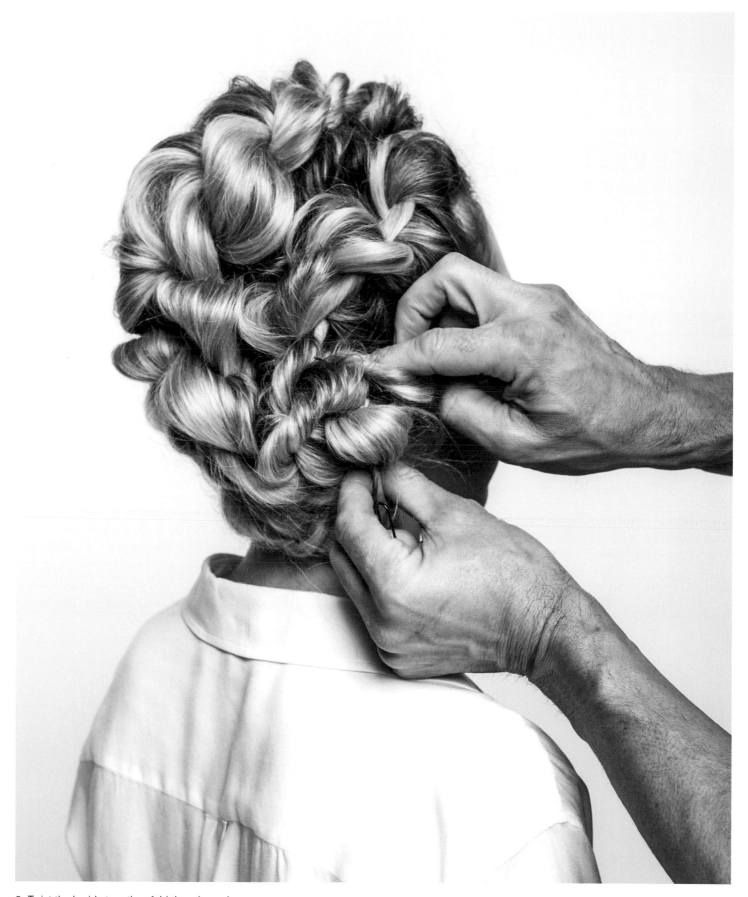

9. Twist the braids together, fold them in, and fasten with hairpins to the anchor point that you created with the bobby pins. Pull and experiment with the style until you are satisfied with the results. Finish with hairspray.

Grecian Tiara

For those of you who want lots of volume, this hairstyle uses rope braids as a tiara to keep height and volume in place. This is an updo that makes a big impression!

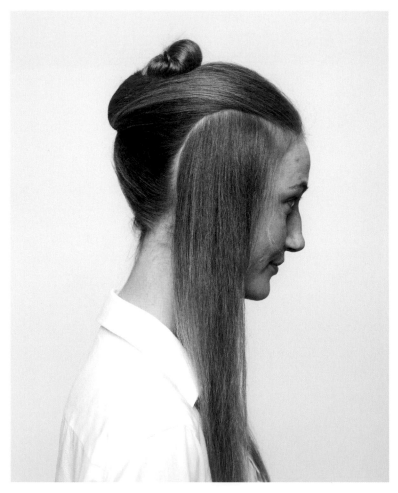

1. Make three sections by drawing two parts, each running along one side of the crown. The parts should go from the hairline in a curve toward the neck.

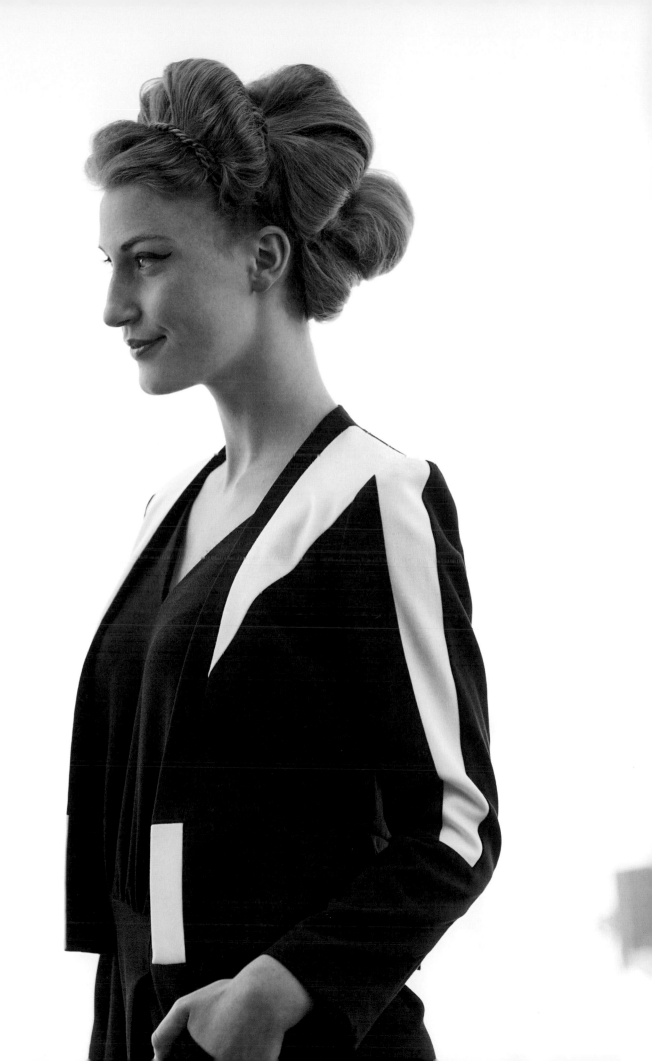

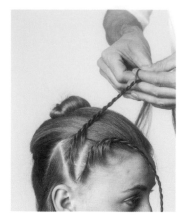

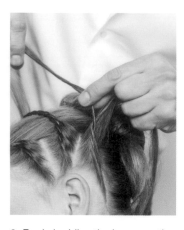

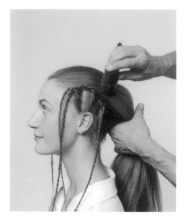

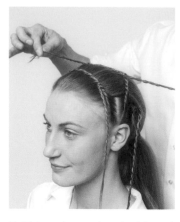

2. Begin by dividing one side section into three smaller sections. You will now make rope braids from each of these smaller sections, starting with the one closest to the face. Make a rope braid by dividing the section into two strands. Twist the right strand inward and switch places by twisting the left strand over the right strand. Add in a little more hair to each strand before you repeat the twist. Continue to twist and switch sides so that a rope-shaped braid is formed. Braid in an upward direction, staying close to the head. Tease the ends to secure the braid. Repeat so that you have three thin braids hanging on each side.

3. Begin braiding the lower section of hair with the same technique as described in step 2. Here you will make just one braid. Braid upward, close to the head. Tease the ends to secure the braid. Repeat steps 2 and 3 on the other side of the head.

4. Unfasten the midsection. Brush the hair straight back. Gather the hair in one hand. Fasten temporarily with an elastic.

5. Pick up the two front braids and twist them together a few times so that they form a tiara over the midsection.

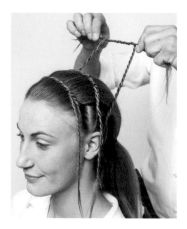

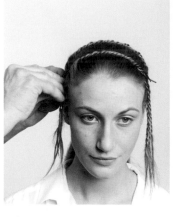

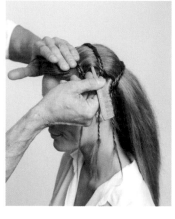

6. Now twist together the other braids in the same way as described in step 5.

7. Secure the braids with short pins.

8. Remove the elastic. Using a rattail comb, lift up the hair between the braids.

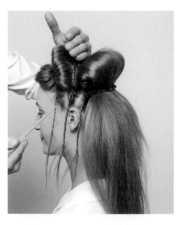

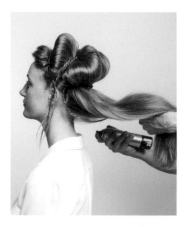

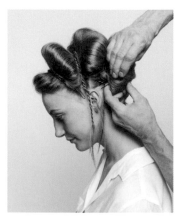

9. When you are satisfied with the amount of volume, secure the hair with long hairpins.

10. Brush the lower part of the hair carefully. Use hairspray on the underside of the hair.

11. Fold in the ends and lay the hair against the head. Fasten with hairpins.

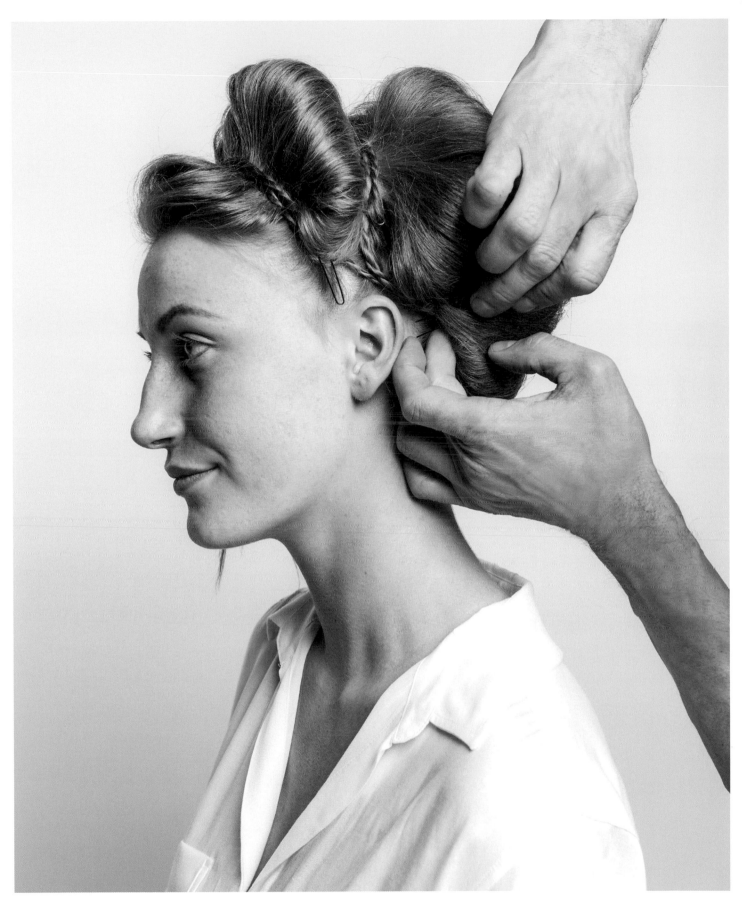

12. Hide the braids under the updo. Fasten with
hairpins. Finish with hairspray.

Margarita Braid

The classic Margarita braid fits any style and works for both everyday and special occasions!

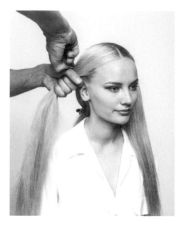

1. Divide the hair into two sections by making a center part down to the nape of the neck. Then divide each section into two equal parts halfway to the back of the head, a front and back section.

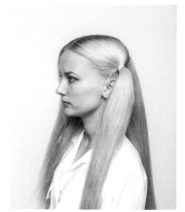

2. Secure each of the front sections in a ponytail above the ear using an elastic band.

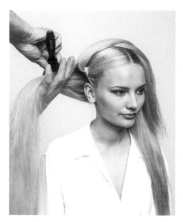

3. Take one of the ponytails and brush upward, toward the other side of the face. Let the ponytail hang toward the other side. Take hold of the lower section on the same side.

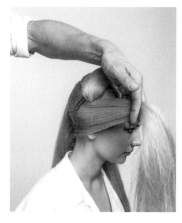

4. Brush the hair straight to the front, toward the eye. Place one hairpin at the part to keep hair in place. Now you will twist the two sections together to make a rope braid.

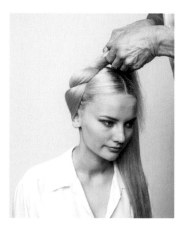

5. Always twist the right strand inward. Switch sides by twisting the left strand over the right one. Continue twisting. Switch sides again and repeat. A rope-shaped braid will take shape. Fasten with an elastic band. Pin the braid temporarily with long hairpins.

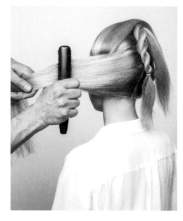

6. Repeat the previous steps, but now on the other side. Take hold of the lower section. Brush the hair straight to the front toward the eye. Use a hairpin at the part to keep hair in its place.

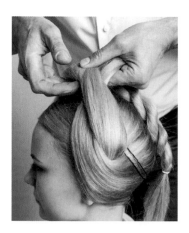

7. Now twist the two ponytails together to make a rope braid using the same technique as described in step 5. Pin the braid temporarily with hairpins.

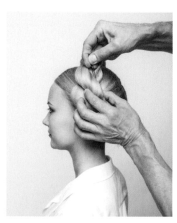

8. Fasten the ends against the base of the ponytails using hairpins and finish with hairspray.

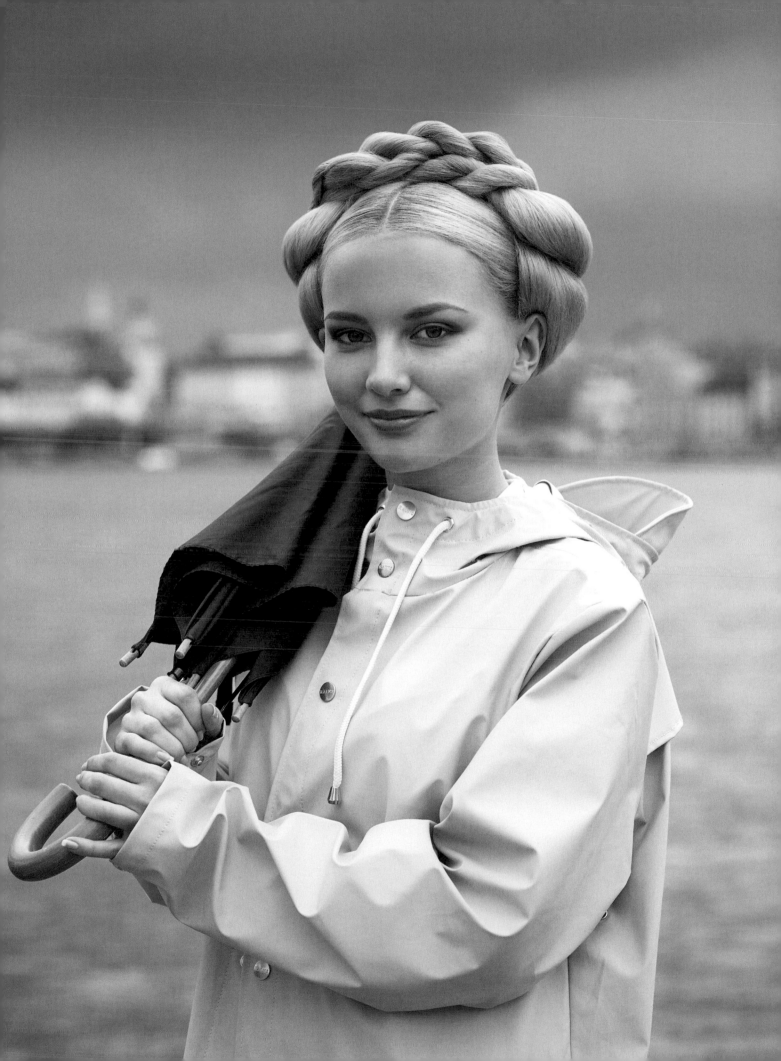

Seaside Tiara

A relaxed hairstyle with a rope braid in the middle, this braid is perfect if you like to wear your hair loose but with a twist!

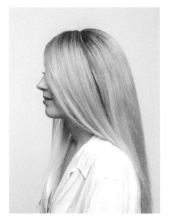

1. Divide hair into three sections. Draw a part from behind one ear across to the other ear, like a tiara.

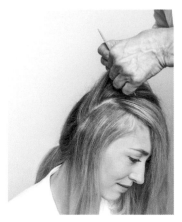

2. Then draw another part from the beginning of the first part, like a point that widens over to the other side of the head.

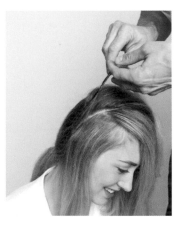

3. Begin braiding the center section. Now you will make a rope braid. Pick up a thin strand and twist it. Pick up one more strand and repeat the twist.

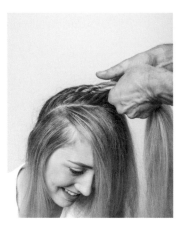

4. Twist the right strand inward. Switch sides by twisting the left strand over the right one. Now twist the right strand inward again. Change places again and repeat so that a rope-shaped braid takes shape.

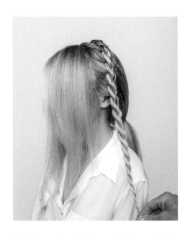

5. Repeat until the entire length is braided. Fasten with an elastic band.

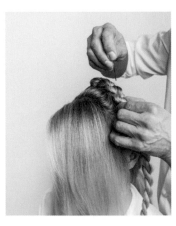

6. Lift the braid on top of the head and fasten with short hairpins.

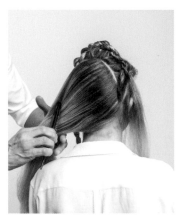

7. Brush the back section to one side, lay it over the shoulder, and finish with hairspray. Also, brush part of the forward section back toward the same shoulder.

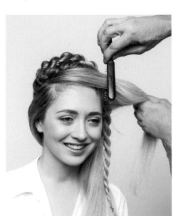

8. Comb the bang section in the shape you desire. Finish with hairspray.

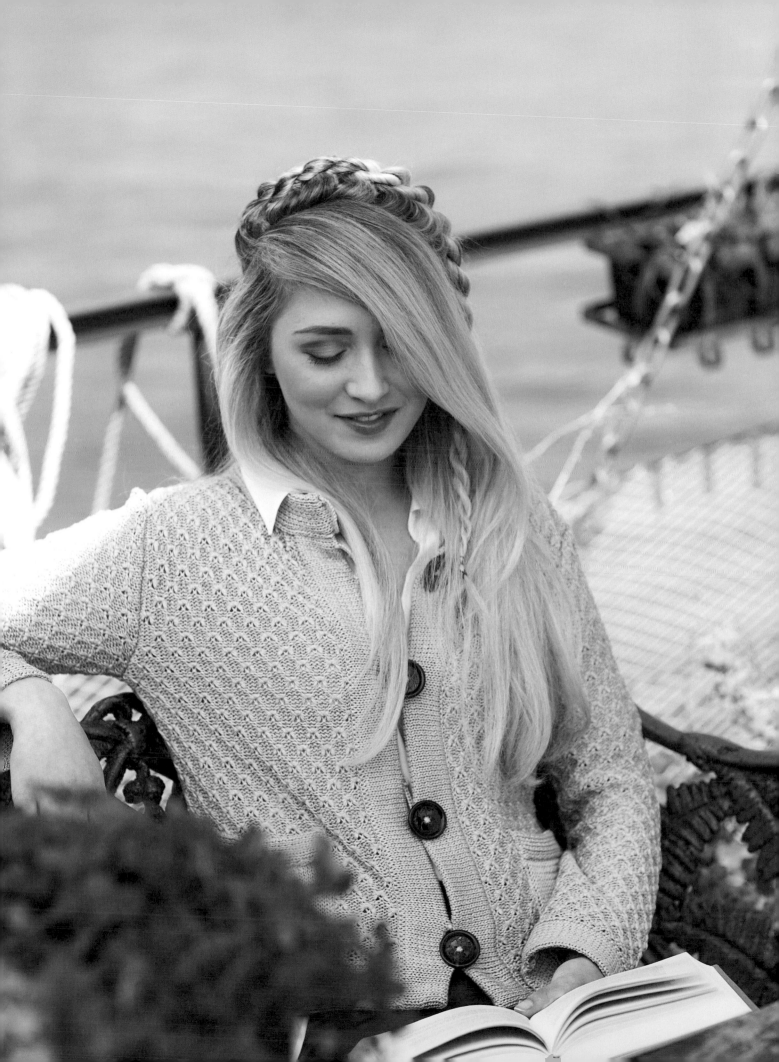

Leia

Both classic and beautiful, with this braid we make a tight bun using two rope braids. It's a perfect braid for people with longer hair!

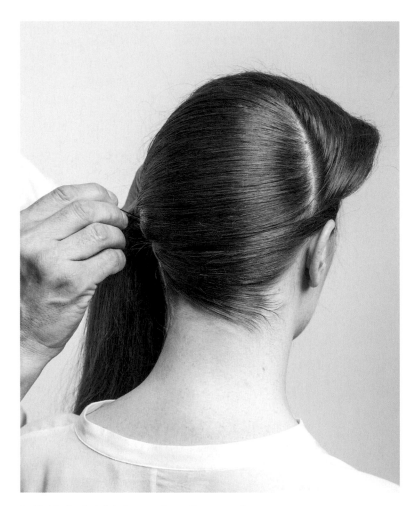

1. Divide the hair into two sections. Draw a part from ear to ear.

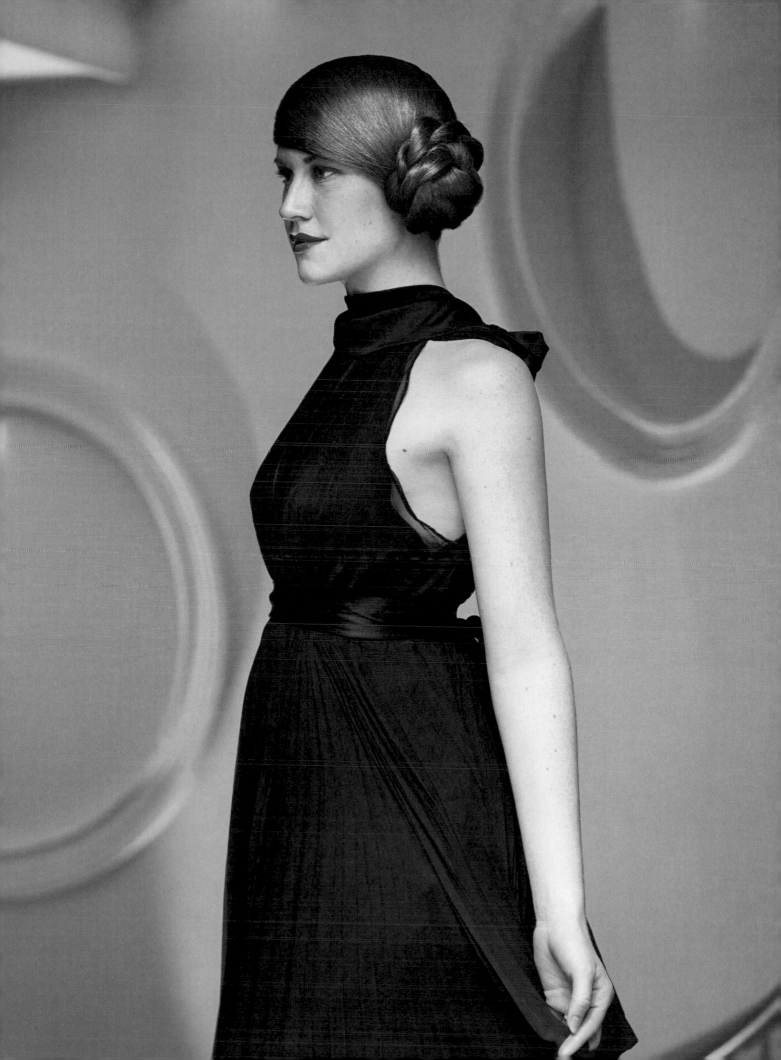

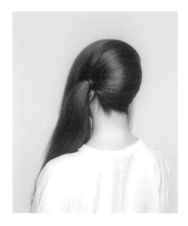

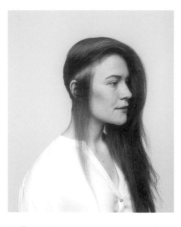

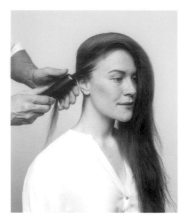

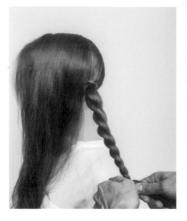

2. Comb the back section tightly to the side and fasten in a ponytail just behind the ear. Fasten with an elastic.

3. From the opposite front section, separate out a strand near the ear.

4. Pull the strand in toward the ponytail. Twist and wrap the strand around the elastic to hide the base of the ponytail. Fasten with a small hairpin. If there isn't enough hair, a strand from the same side as the ponytail can be used.

5. Begin braiding the ponytail. Here you will make a rope braid. Divide the hair into two parts. Always twist the right strand inward. Switch sides by twisting the left strand over of the right one. Continue twisting, switch places again and repeat so that a rope-shaped braid is formed. Twist the entire length and fasten with an elastic.

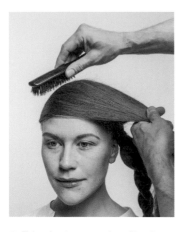

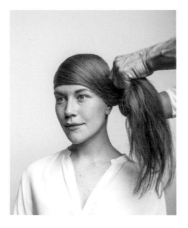

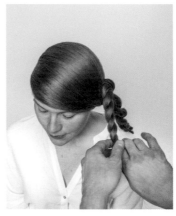

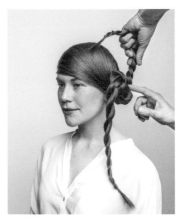

6. Take the front section. Brush the hair toward the same side as the braid, close to the head and across the forehead, like a hat. Use an extra long hairpin for support.

7. Wrap the hair once around the base of the ponytail.

8. Make another rope braid in the same way as in step 5. Fasten with an elastic.

9. Now you will make a bun at the side of the head using both rope braids. Wrap the back braid forward toward the face. Fasten with hairpins, using the base of the ponytail as an anchor. Then wrap the front braid back toward the neck. Fasten with hairpins to the base of the ponytail.

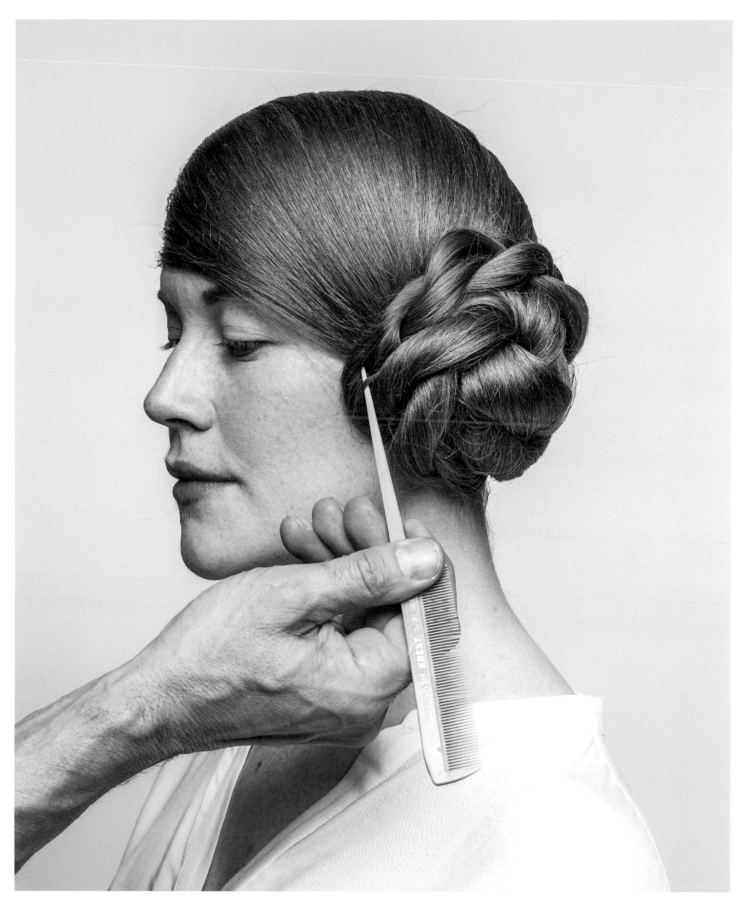

10. Fix any wisps that may stick out from the
bang section and finish with hairspray.

Messy Rope Bun

Twisting the hair can be an alternative to braiding. It gives a similar effect but is both easier and faster. Hair is twisted upward and meets in a messy bun.

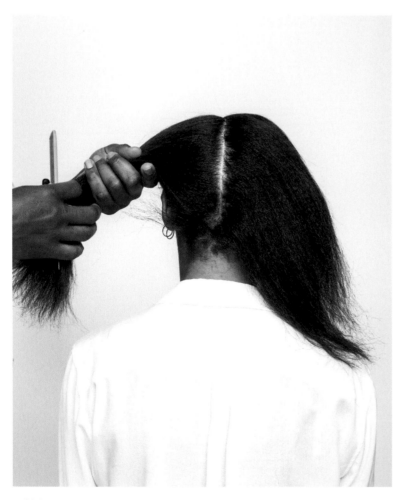

1. Make a center part that runs in a straight line from the forehead to the neck.

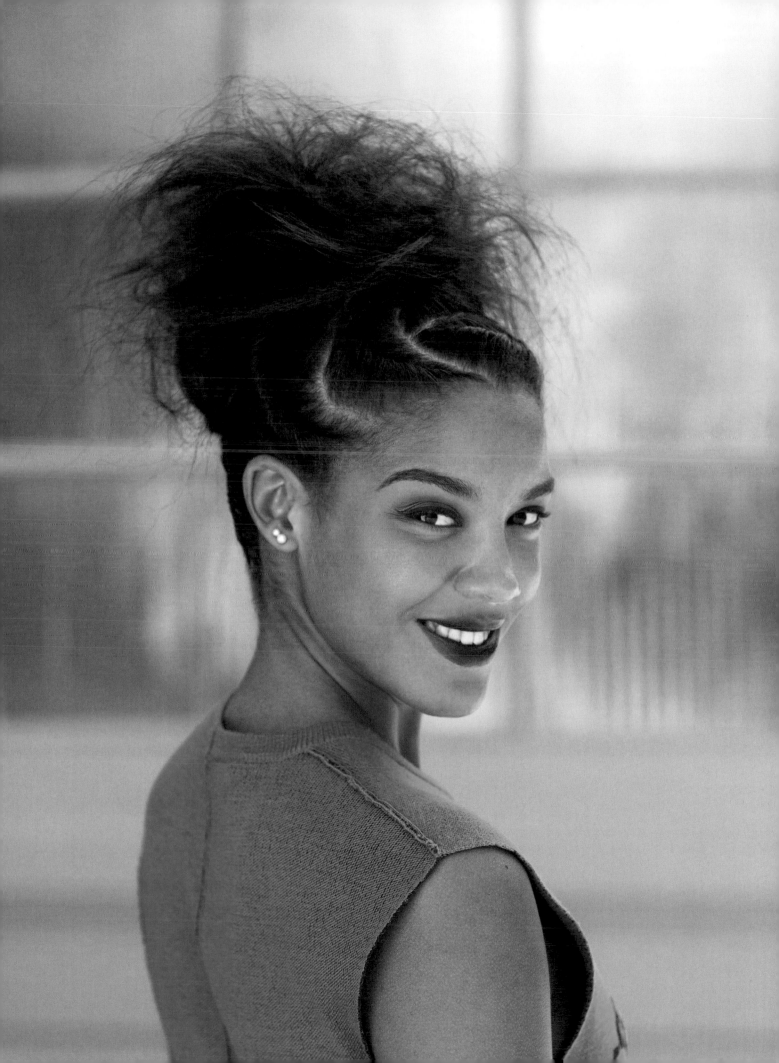

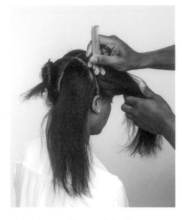

2. Make another part that runs from ear to ear. Now you have divided the hair into four sections.

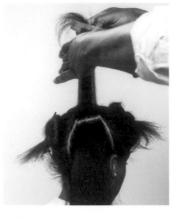

3. Using a rattail comb, take out a strand of hair from each of the four sections. This fifth section functions as the center point. Fasten the first four sections with hair clips.

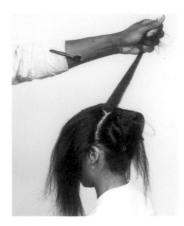

4. Gather up the hair at the center of the crown, as close to the head as possible.

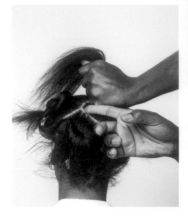

5. Make a ponytail using the hair from the four sections, and fasten with an elastic band. Make sure the ponytail is stable, since it will be the anchor point for the entire hairdo.

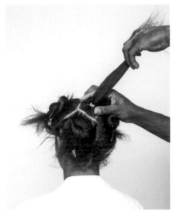

6. Twist the hair in the front section. This section will be divided into three smaller parts, of which the one closest to the part will be a smaller section. Trace a soft S with the tail of the comb in order to make a shaped part.

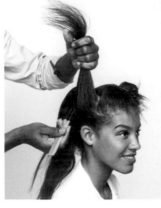

7. Begin twisting from the hairline, always moving toward the center point. For best results, use high-control hairspray. Spray the hair as you twist, so that the hair is wet with spray.

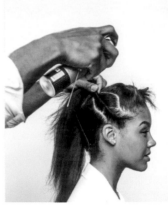

8. Use small pinching movements as you twist in order to catch all the hairs. Secure the twisted strand using two crossed bobby pins at the base of the ponytail.

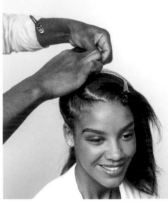

9. Repeat step 7 with the upper section that starts at the temple. Divide this one with an S shape before you twist. Secure with hairspray and fasten with two crossed pins at the base of the ponytail. The two twisted strands meet at the base of the ponytail.

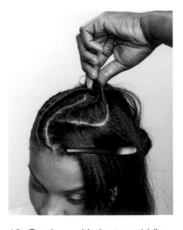

10. Continue with the top middle section. Twist this one also as in step 7 and secure at the base of the ponytail.

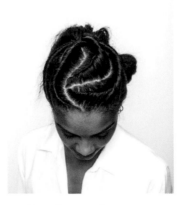

11. Have the parts form a wave pattern with the rope sections pointing toward the base of the ponytail. Continue to repeat the twisting at the front section of the bangs. Fasten at the base and secure with hairspray.

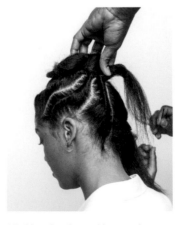

12. Now begin working on the two lower sections. Divide the hair into three equally big parts. Twist the three parts in the same way as in step 7, up toward the midpoint. Secure with hairpins.

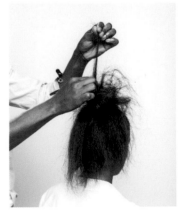

13. Finally, start making the bun. Take one strand at a time and lightly tease with fingers down toward the center point. Repeat until all the hair is teased.

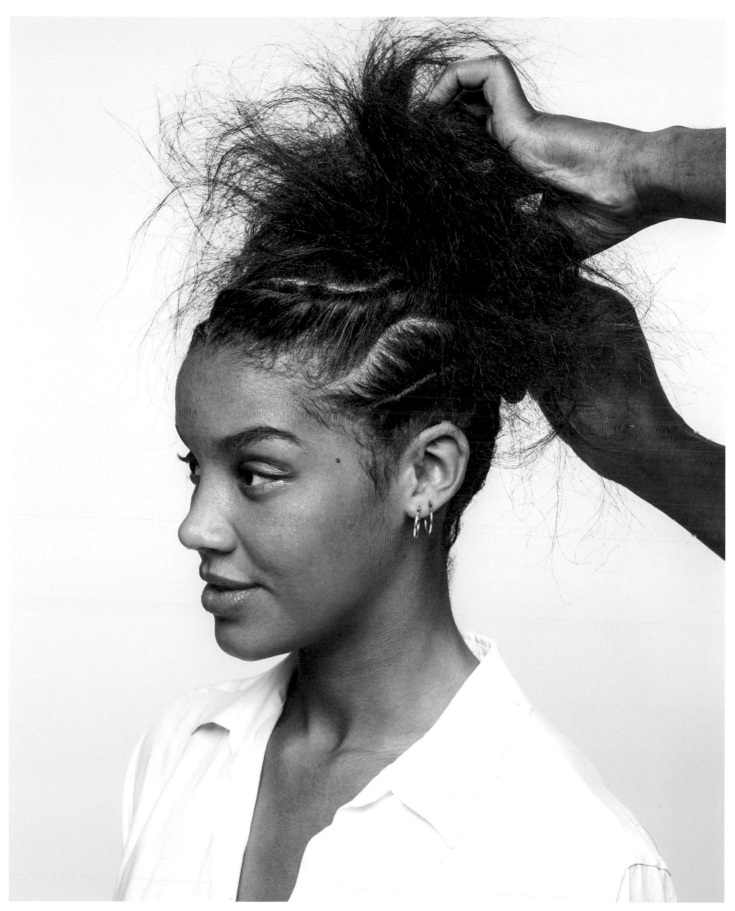

14. Use long hairpins to secure the hair, rotate the pin and fasten to the midpoint. Use as many pins as you need to achieve a stable and secure style.

Avatar

In this hairstyle we mix soft rope braids with teased ends to create stylish contrasts. This is a hairstyle that makes a statement!

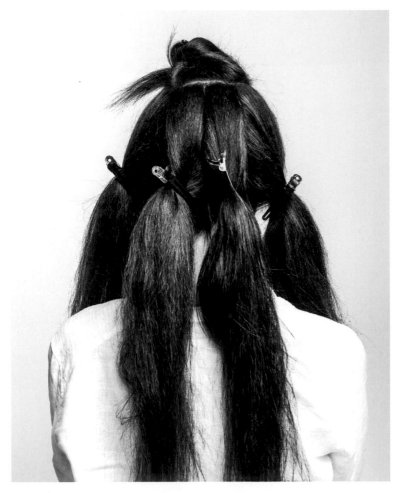

1. Divide hair into five sections. First, separate the crown hair and fasten it out of the way with a hair clip. Then divide the lower section into three equal parts. Divide the middle of these sections into two smaller parts. Fasten with hair clips.

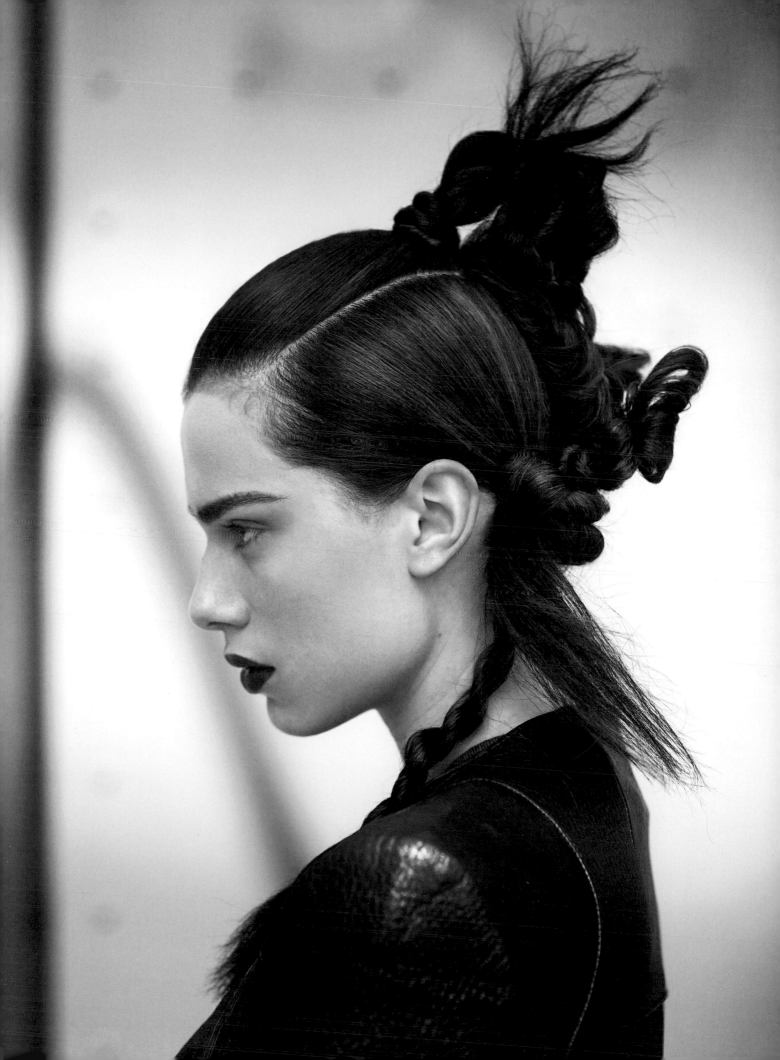

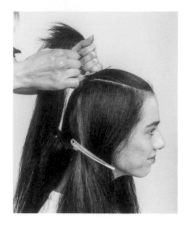

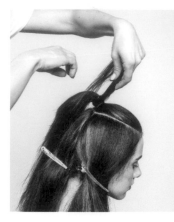

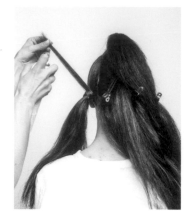

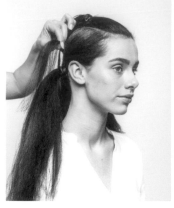

2. Gather crown hair and brush it back, close to the head. Use a shine cream as you work with the hair. Fasten the ponytail with an elastic, making sure that it is securely fastened.

3. Take one strand from the ponytail and twist it around the ponytail base to hide the elastic. Fasten with a small hairpin.

4. With one of the side sections, brush the hair back, close to the head. Make a ponytail and secure with an elastic. Remove one strand from the ponytail, twist it around the base to hide the elastic, and fasten with a small hairpin.

5. Continue to the other side section and repeat step 4.

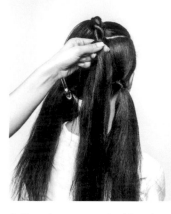

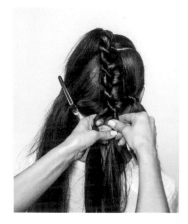

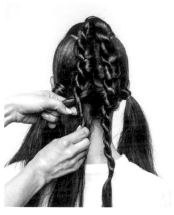

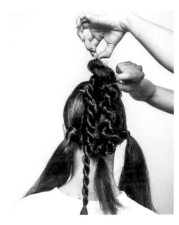

6. To make two rope braids using the crown hair, divide the ponytail into two sections. Divide one of the sections into two strands. Braid toward the back. Always twist the right strand inward. Switch sides by crossing the left strand over the right one. Twist the right strand. Repeat until you have a rope braid.

7. When the braid meets the lower section of hair, begin integrating hair from this lower section into the rope braid as you work. Leave 4 inches of the length unbraided.

8. Now braid the other section in the same way as in steps 6 and 7.

9. Pull at the braids with your fingers to add volume. Begin at the bottom and work your way up.

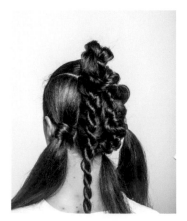

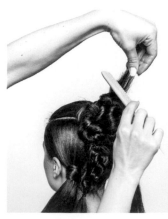

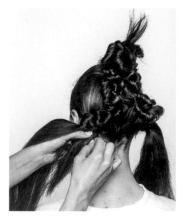

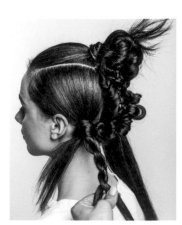

10. Create height in the braids using hairpins, two or three pins in each braid.

11. If you want, you can let parts of the hair stick out of the braid. Tease lightly with a comb and set with hairspray.

12. Fasten ends to the side with hairpins so that the ends point forward, toward the face.

13. Now braid the side sections using the same technique as described in step 6.

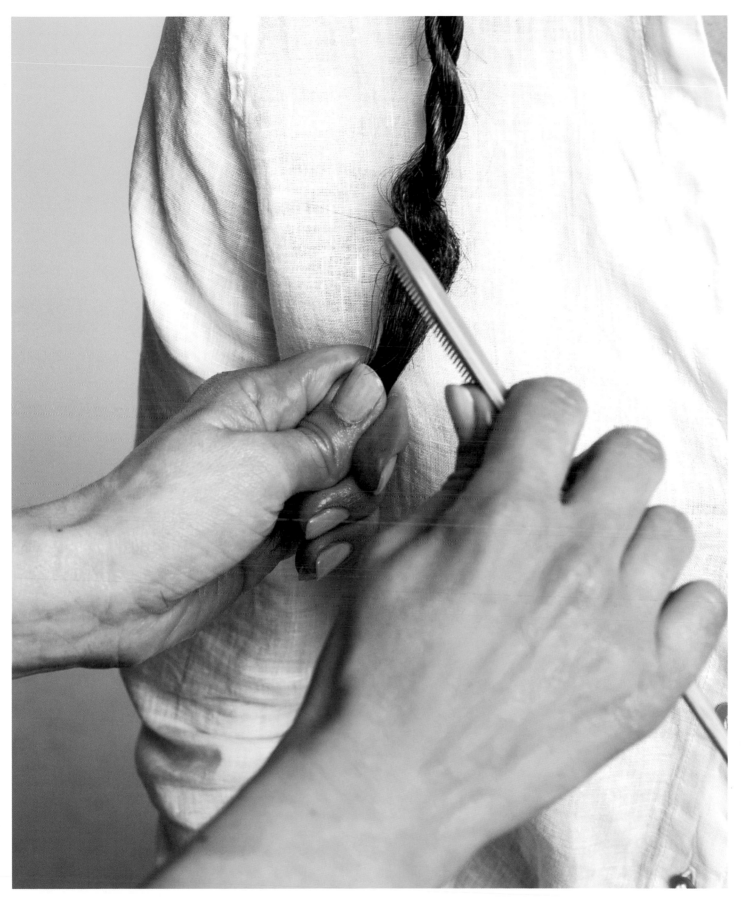

14. Instead of fastening with an elastic, tease the
ends to keep the braids in place.

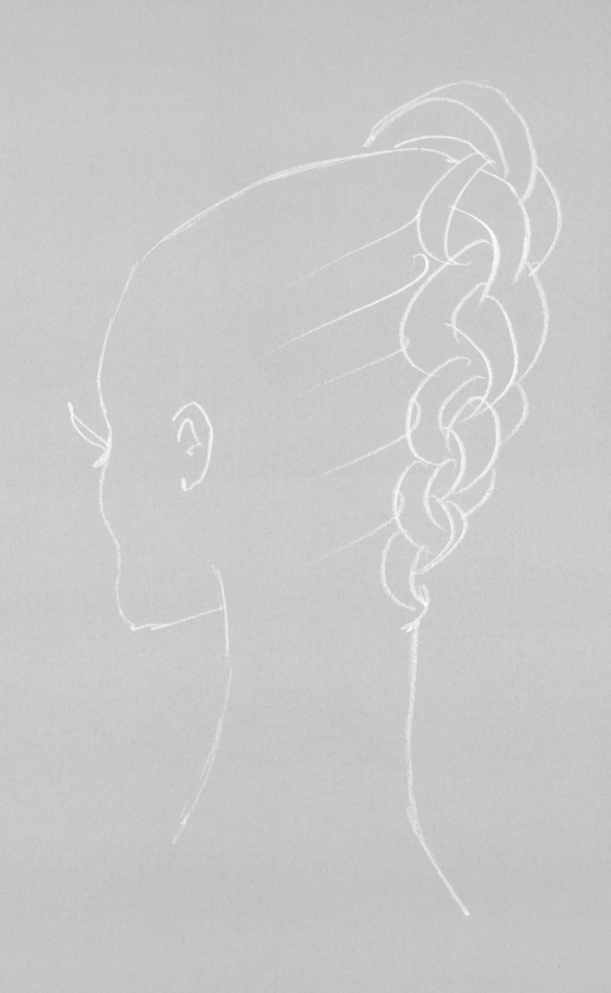

Playful Braids

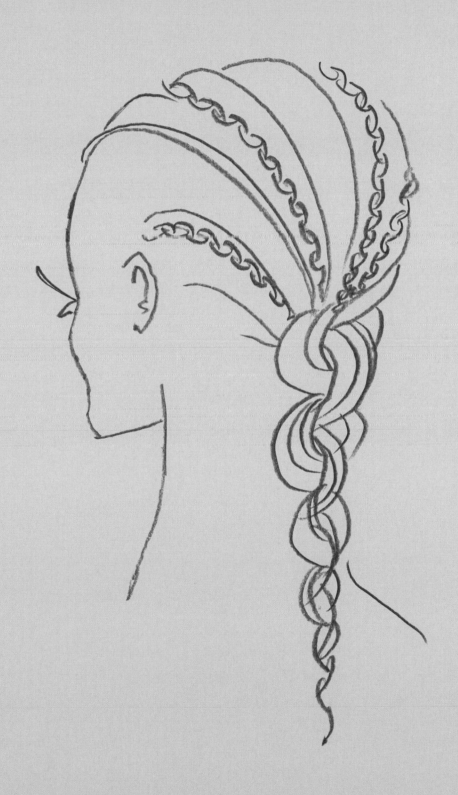

Chain Braid

This hairstyle requires an extra pair of hands. The stylish chain braid is a fun alternative to the rope braid.

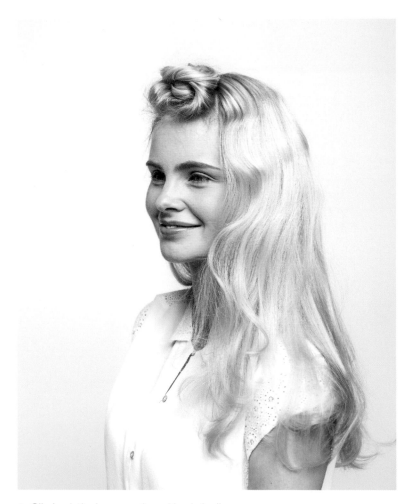

1. Clip back the bang section with a hair clip.

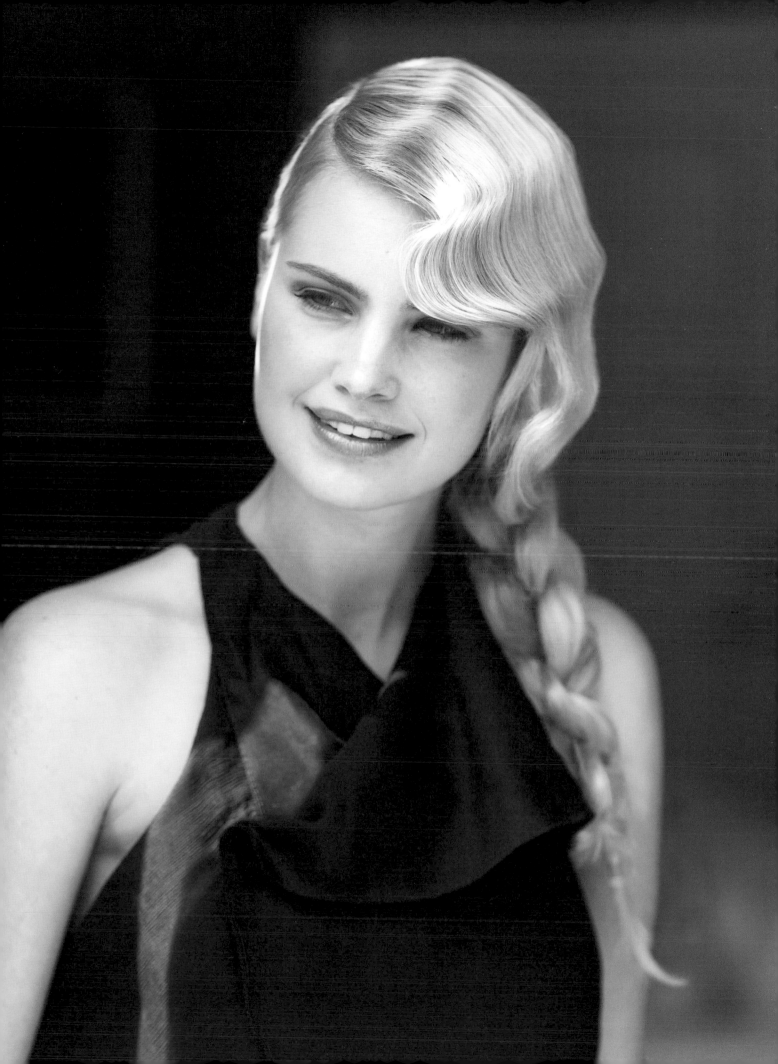

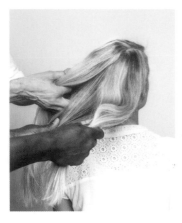

2. Sweep the rest of the hair to one side of the face. Divide into two equal parts.

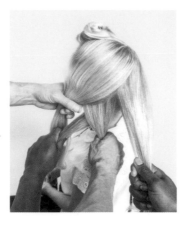

3. Divide each section into two smaller sections, upper and lower.

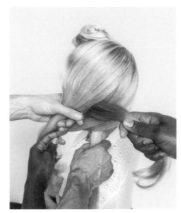

4. Each person will hold two smaller sections, one from the upper part and one from the lower part. You will take turns braiding.

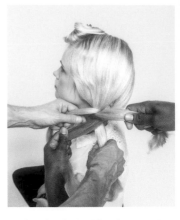

5. Now begin braiding by crossing the sections, alternating horizontal and vertical crossings.

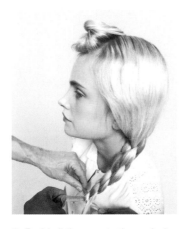

6. Braid all the way to the end of the hair. Fasten with an elastic.

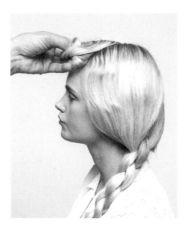

7. Release the bang section and brush it smoothly toward the braid. Curl the bangs if you wish.

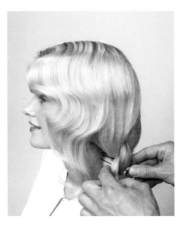

8. Now you will integrate the bangs into the braid. Push an extra long hairpin through one loop of the braid.

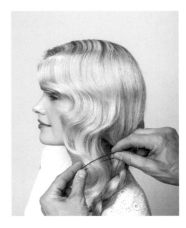

9. Use another hairpin to catch the bang section.

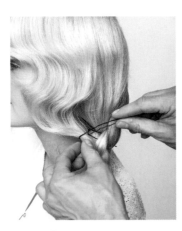

10. Pull the hairpin with the bang section through the hairpin inserted in the braid in order to integrate the bangs and make them melt into the braid.

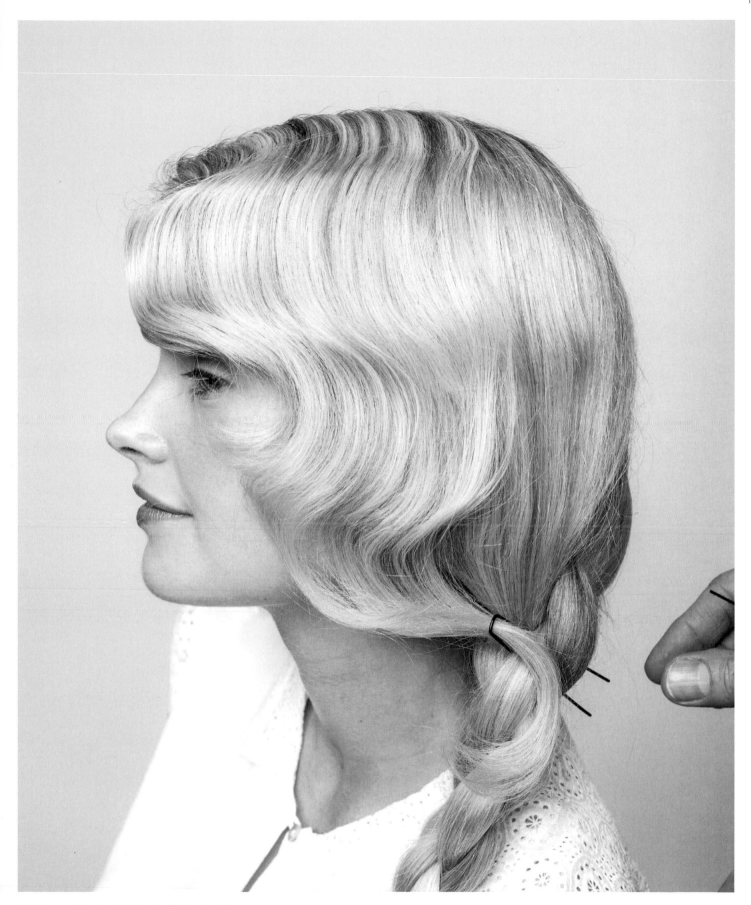

11. Now pull the hairpin inserted in the braid down through the braid in order to fasten the bangs. Secure with a hairpin. Use hairspray for stability.

Mixed-Hat Braid

Combine different types of braids within one hairstyle to create an exciting and modern look! Here we combine a French braid, a knotted braid, and a Dutch braid in one single style.

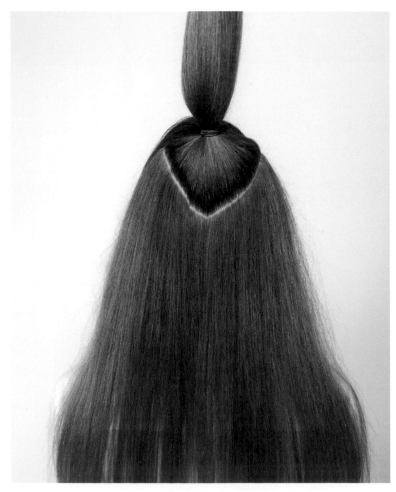

1. Gather the hair at the back of the head into a ponytail by drawing a V-shaped part that points down toward the neck. Secure hair in a ponytail using an elastic. Twist the ponytail together with the bang section and temporarily pin out of the way with a hairpin.

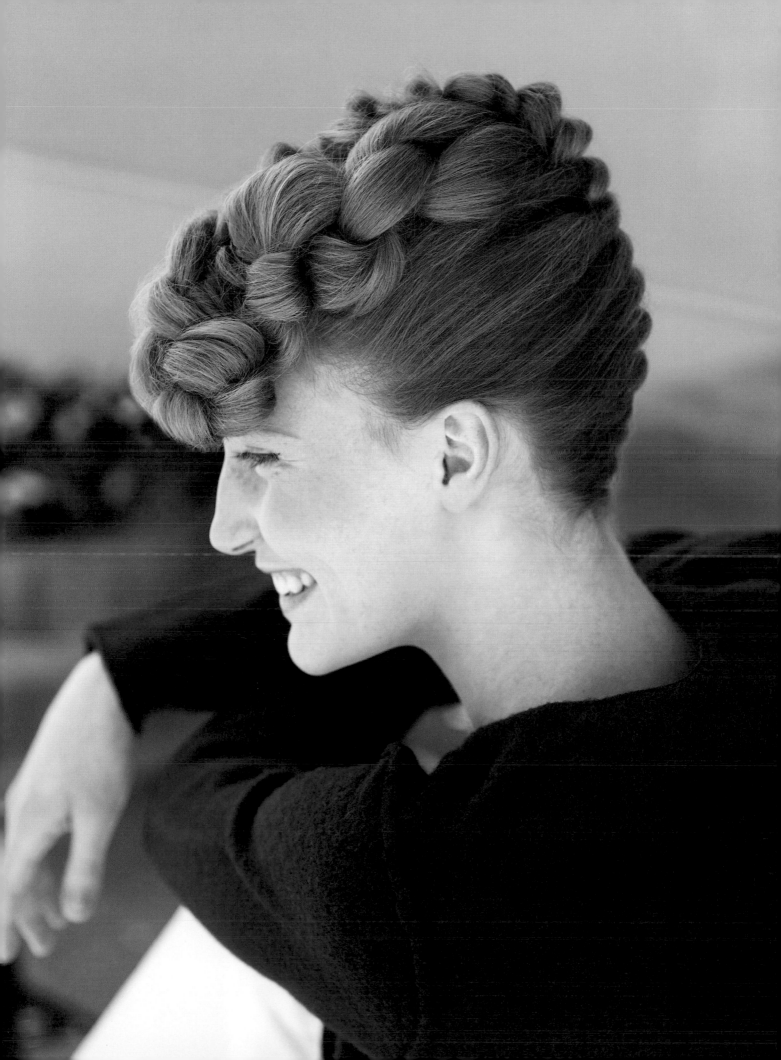

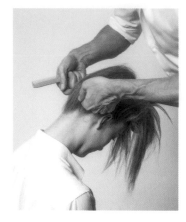

2. Gather the lower section of hair and brush it upward. Spray with hairspray and continue brushing upward to achieve a smooth surface.

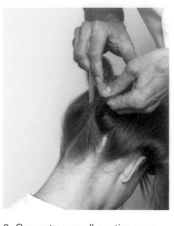

3. Separate a small section near the neck, divide into three strands and make a French braid. Make one round of a basic braid. Then add in a new strand of hair from the outside with each new crossing.

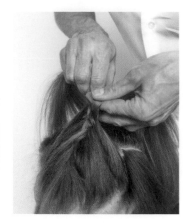

4. Alternate right and left sides, adding in new strands to each section of hair. The braid will run up the center of the head toward the crown. Repeat until the entire length of hair is braided. Fasten with a thin elastic.

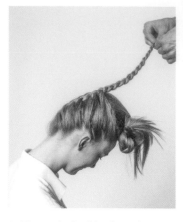

5. Pin up the braid using a large hairpin.

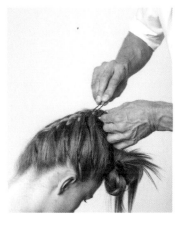

6. Tuck in any wisps at the sides, using the end of a comb. Use hairspray as you work to achieve a smooth surface.

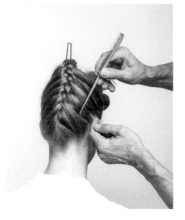

7. Now begin braiding the ponytail in a knotted braid. Divide into two equal parts. Make a regular knot.

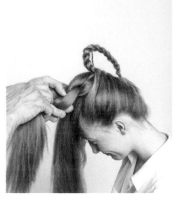

8. Continue knotting the entire length. Fasten with an elastic. Put the knotted braid to one side.

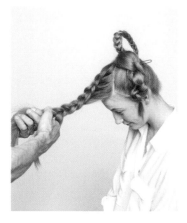

9. Brush the hair in the front section and divide it into three strands to make a Dutch braid. Make one round of a basic braid, where the side strands are crossed under the center strand. With each new crossing, add a new strand from the outside. Alternate right and left sides until the entire length is braided. Fasten with an elastic.

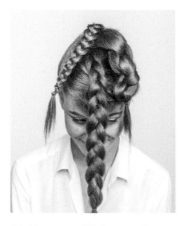

10. Now you will bring together the three different braids. Move all the braids forward toward the face.

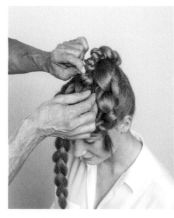

11. Pull at the French braid for a more relaxed feeling.

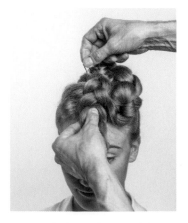

12. Fold in the ends toward the center of the head and fasten with a hairpin.

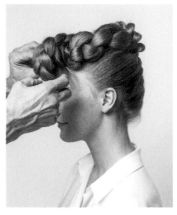

13. Attach the knotted braid by folding in the ends. Fasten with pins.

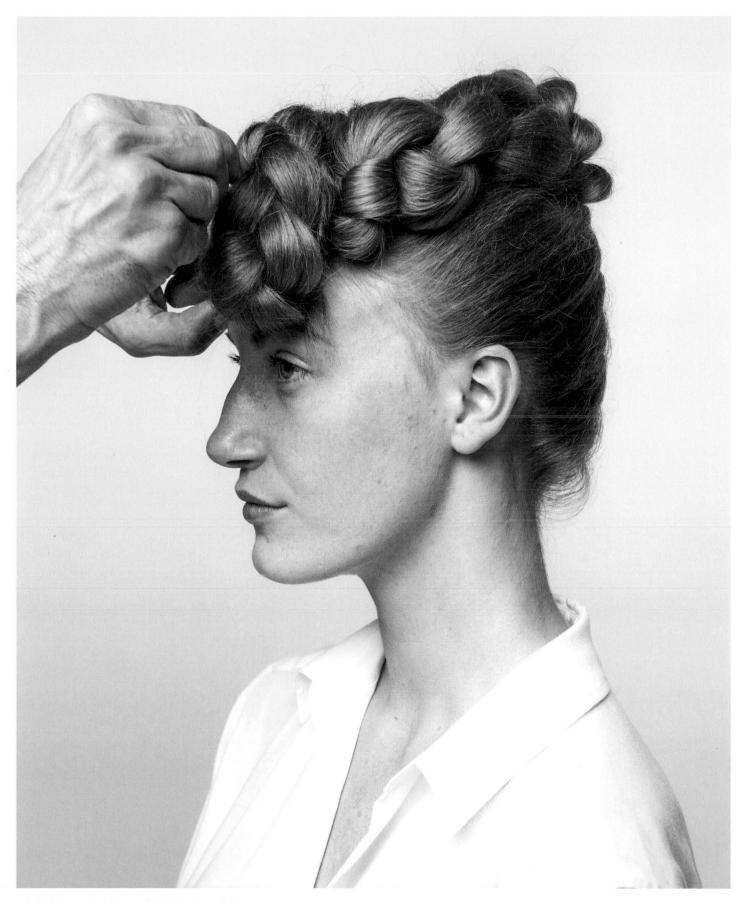

14. Finish by attaching the Dutch braid. Roll the ends in and fasten with hairpins. Set the hairstyle with hairspray.

Street Braid

Braid the hair away from the face and let it hang loose down the back.
The street braid is elegant, modern, and goes with any look.

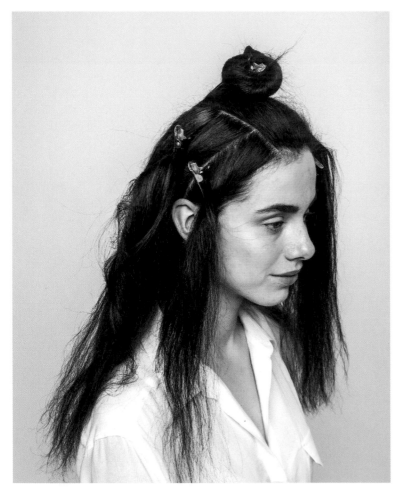

1. Divide the hair into six sections. Separate one
narrow section at the crown, about 2.5 inches wide.
Fasten out of the way with a hair clip. Separate out
two sections on each side of the face, about 1 inch
wide. The remaining hair will be the sixth section.

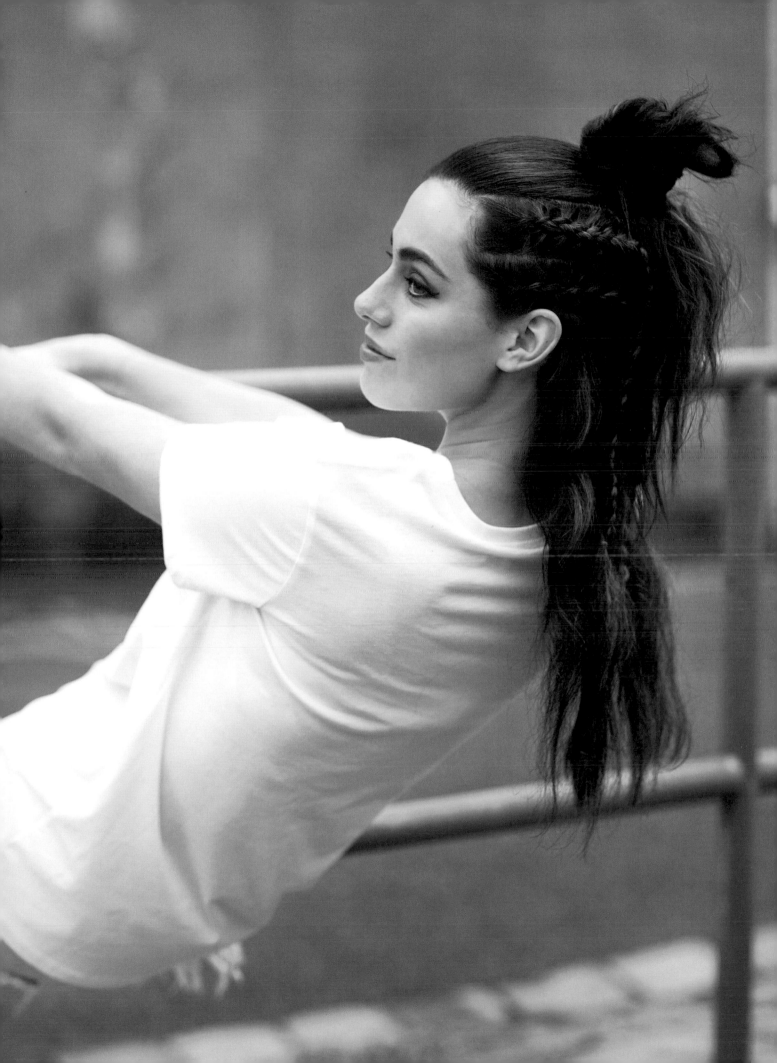

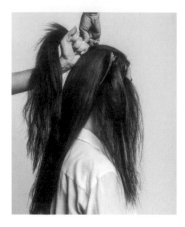

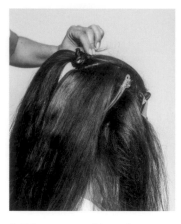

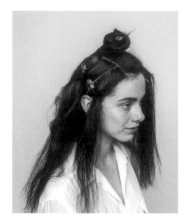

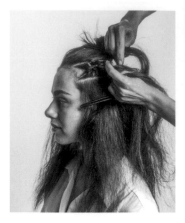

2. Comb the crown section smooth. Gather hair into a ponytail and fasten with an elastic.

3. Take one strand from the ponytail and twist it. Wrap the strand around the base of the ponytail to conceal the elastic. Fasten with a small hairpin. Put up the ponytail with a hair clip.

4. Now comb through one of the upper front sections.

5. To make a Dutch braid, divide the section into three strands. Make one round of a regular braid, where the side strands are crossed under the center strand. Then add in a new strand of hair from outside with each new crossing.

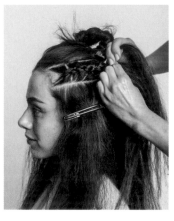

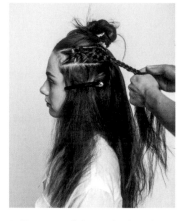

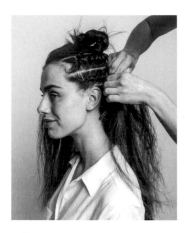

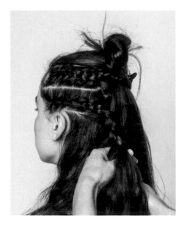

6. Alternate right and left sides, adding in new strands of hair to each section. Braid toward the back, staying close to the head.

7. Repeat until the entire length is braided. Fasten with an elastic. Pin the braid up temporarily using a hairpin.

8. Repeat steps 5 and 6 for the lower front section.

9. As you make this braid, you can integrate hair from the back section so that the braid becomes thicker. Fasten with an elastic.

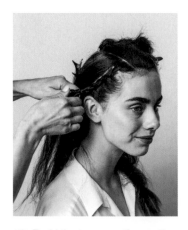

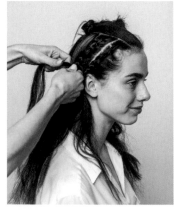

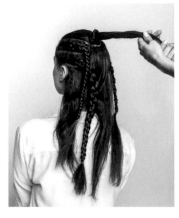

10. Braid the lower section on the other side of the head in the same way as in steps 5 and 6. Braid down toward the lower part of the ear and fasten with an elastic.

11. Braid the upper section in the same way as in steps 5 and 6. On this side, you will only braid half the length.

12. Twist the ponytail up on the crown.

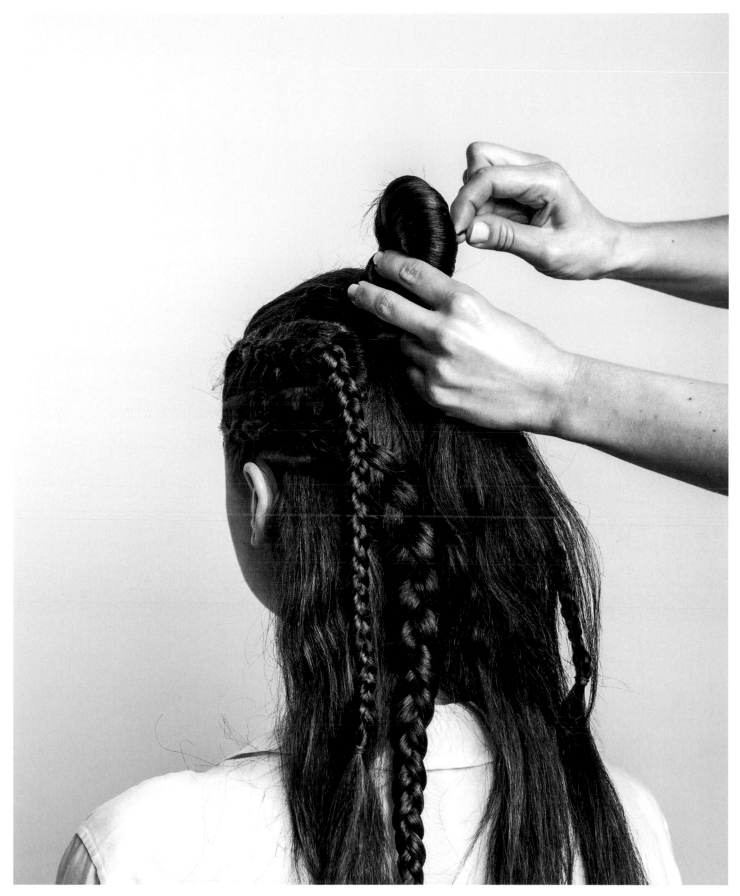

13. Wrap the ponytail around the elastic and let the ends hang out. Fasten with pins. Pull the hair forward and up to give the hairstyle more height. Finish with hairspray.

Pinecone Braid

An updo with a little something extra, this simple four-way braid becomes an elegant style when you play with the shape. Even a beginner can master this braid!

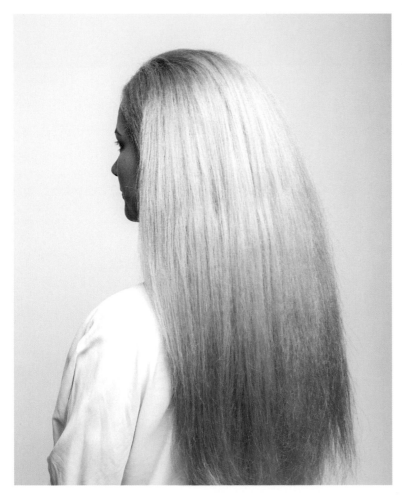

1. Gather all the hair to the back.

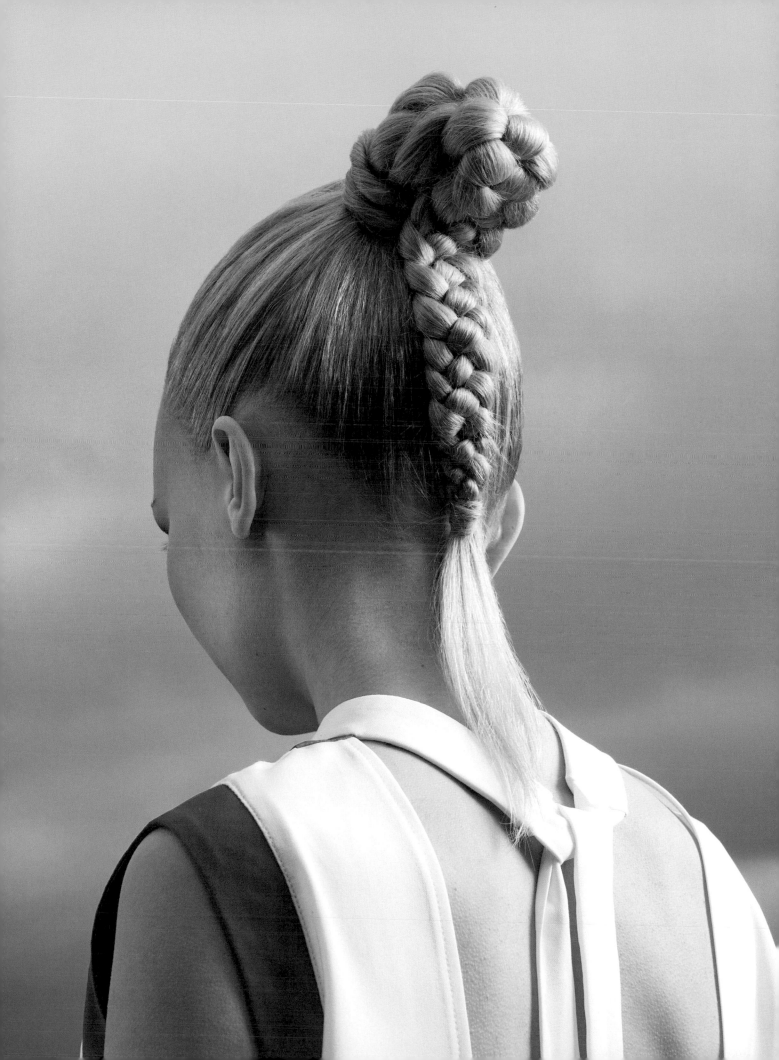

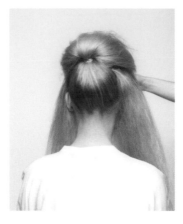

2. Separate the hair at the neck, forming a section from ear to ear straight up toward the crown. Pull this lower section of hair upward into a ponytail and fasten with an elastic.

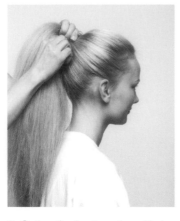

3. Gather the front section of hair. Brush it in toward the ponytail, but don't pull the hair as tightly against the head. Let this hair remain looser to create more volume. Now fasten the upper hair into a ponytail along with the first ponytail by using an elastic.

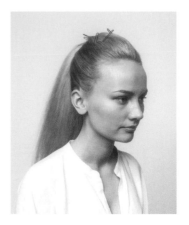

4. Lift the front hair using a rattail comb to create volume. Insert bobby pins as supports in the hair, using them like a fence around the shape to keep it in place.

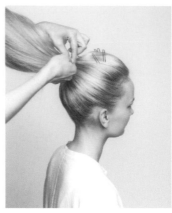

5. Take one strand from the ponytail and twist it. Wrap the strand around the base of the ponytail to conceal the elastic. Fasten with a small pin.

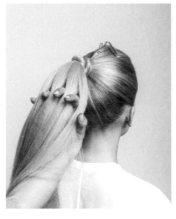

6. Divide the ponytail into four sections using your fingers.

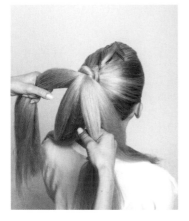

7. Make a four-strand braid with the ponytail. Braid loosely at the beginning. Make one round as a regular three-strand braid, beginning with the left outer strand. Let the right strand wait. Cross the strand over the center strand.

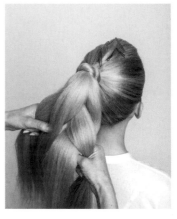

8. After this crossover, now take the right strand and bring it in to the center from underneath. Continue with a new three-strand crossing and then take the leftmost strand and bring it to the center from underneath.

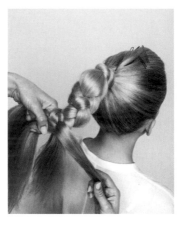

9. Braid the entire ponytail and fasten with an elastic.

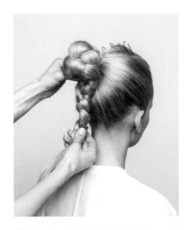

10. Fasten the braid to the base of the ponytail using hairpins.

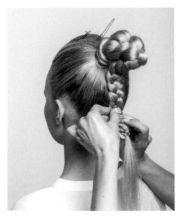

11. Continue fastening the braid against the head using pins.

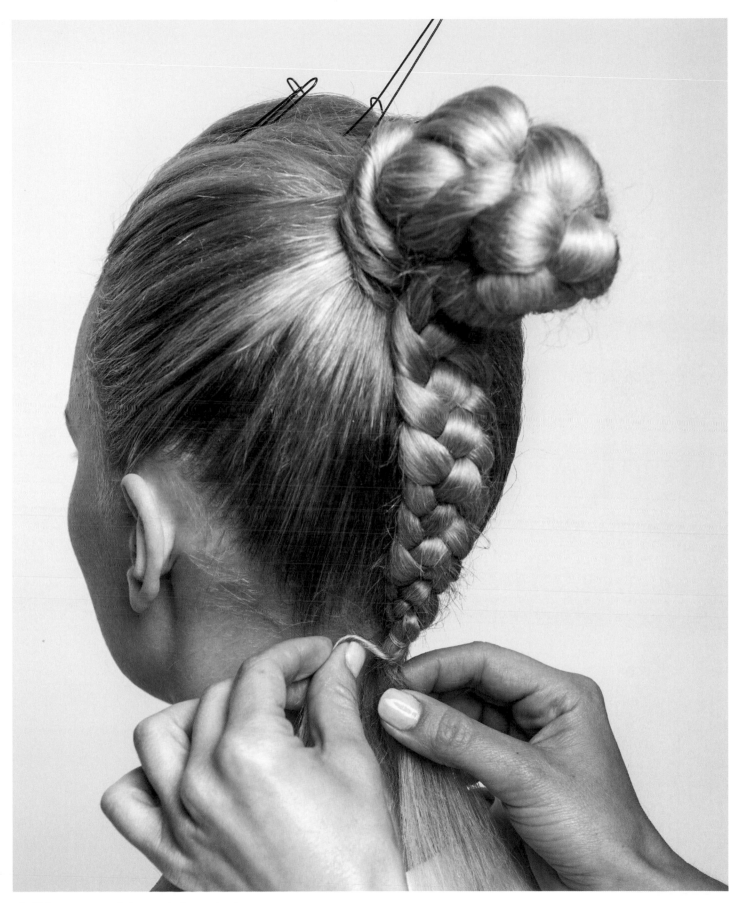

12. Pick up one strand close to the lower elastic, twist it and wrap around the base to conceal the elastic. Take out the bobby pins at the crown. Finish with hairspray.

Basket Braid

A true classic, the basket braid gives you a beautiful woven pattern. Combine it here with loose ends for a relaxed feel.

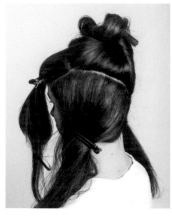

1. Divide the hair into four sections. Separate the bang section. Then draw a V-shaped part down toward the neck. Pin the crown hair with a hair clip. Divide the lower section of hair into two parts.

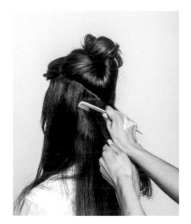

2. Begin working with the left lower section. Tease close to the part to create volume.

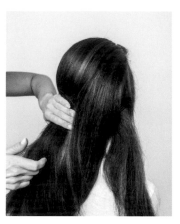

3. Release the crown hair and pin it down in line with the teasing underneath.

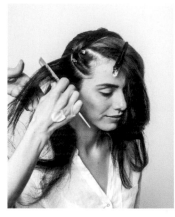

4. Now return to the right lower section. Take out smaller sections about .5 to .75 inches wide. Fasten with small hair clips. Use shine cream as you work with the strands.

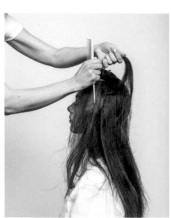

5. Unfasten the bang section. Repeat step 4. Now you can begin making your basket braid.

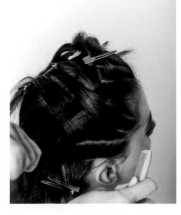

6. You have divided the hair into strands that are both horizontal and vertical. The horizontal strands will be woven together with the vertical ones.

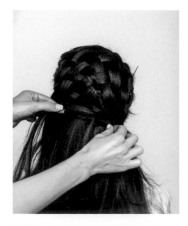

7. Thread the horizontal strands one by one across the vertical strands, crossing alternately over and under them. Repeat, wrapping the woven strands over and knotting the remaining ends. Fasten with hairpins. Finish with hairspray.

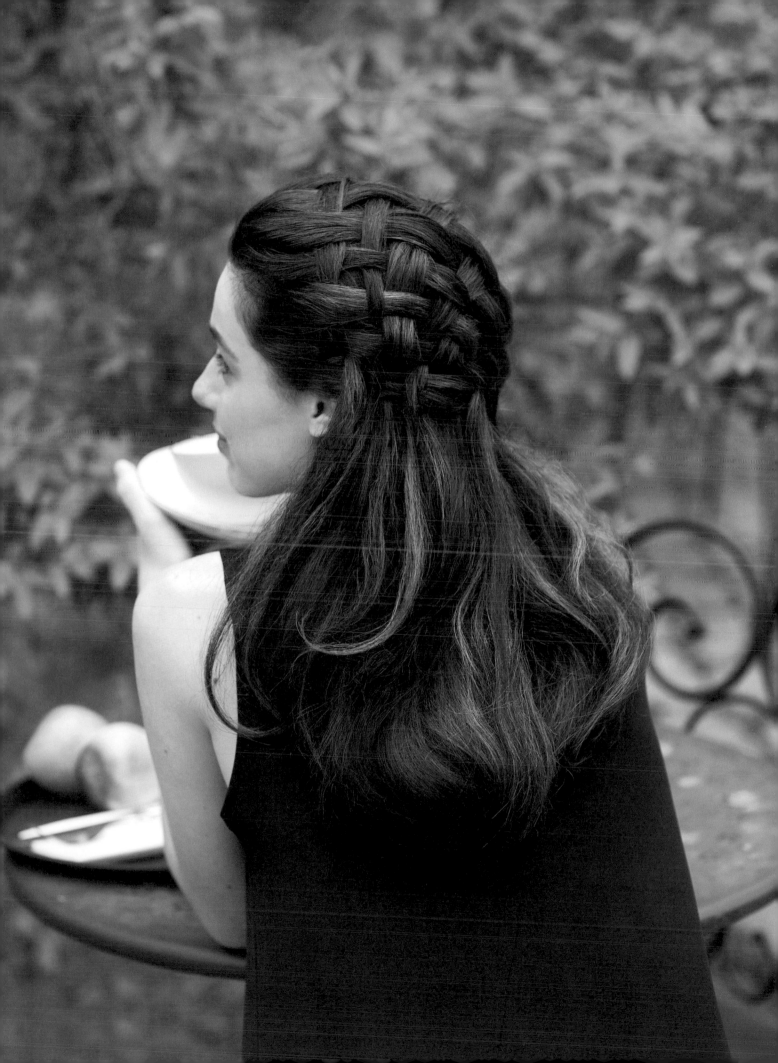

Jasmine

By linking several braids together, you can make a substantial hairstyle that gets attention. It looks advanced but is easy to make!

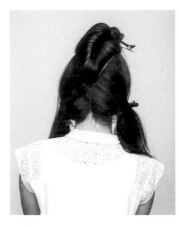

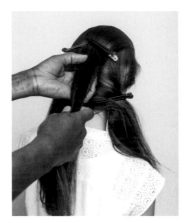

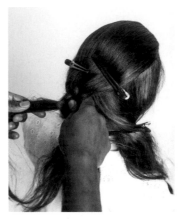

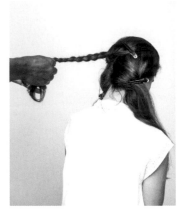

1. Divide the hair into three sections by drawing a sharply V-shaped part down toward the neck. Fasten out of the way with hair clips.

2. Begin with the middle section. Fasten two hair clips at the top of the crown to keep hair in place as you braid a five-part braid.

3. Divide the midsection into five strands. Braid with the three right-most strands by making one round of a three-part braid, beginning with the outermost right strand. Continue by braiding with the three leftmost strands, beginning with the outermost left strand. Repeat the steps using the three right strands.

4. Braid the entire length and fasten with an elastic.

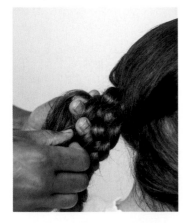

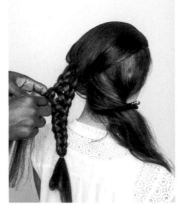

5. Continue with the side section and make a three-part braid. Before you make the second crossing, pull one of the strands through the center braid to link together with the five-part braid in the midsection.

6. Continue braiding. Always pull a new strand through the center braid before each crossover. This will link the braids together. Repeat in the same way on the opposite side. Fasten the big braid with an elastic. Finish with hairspray.

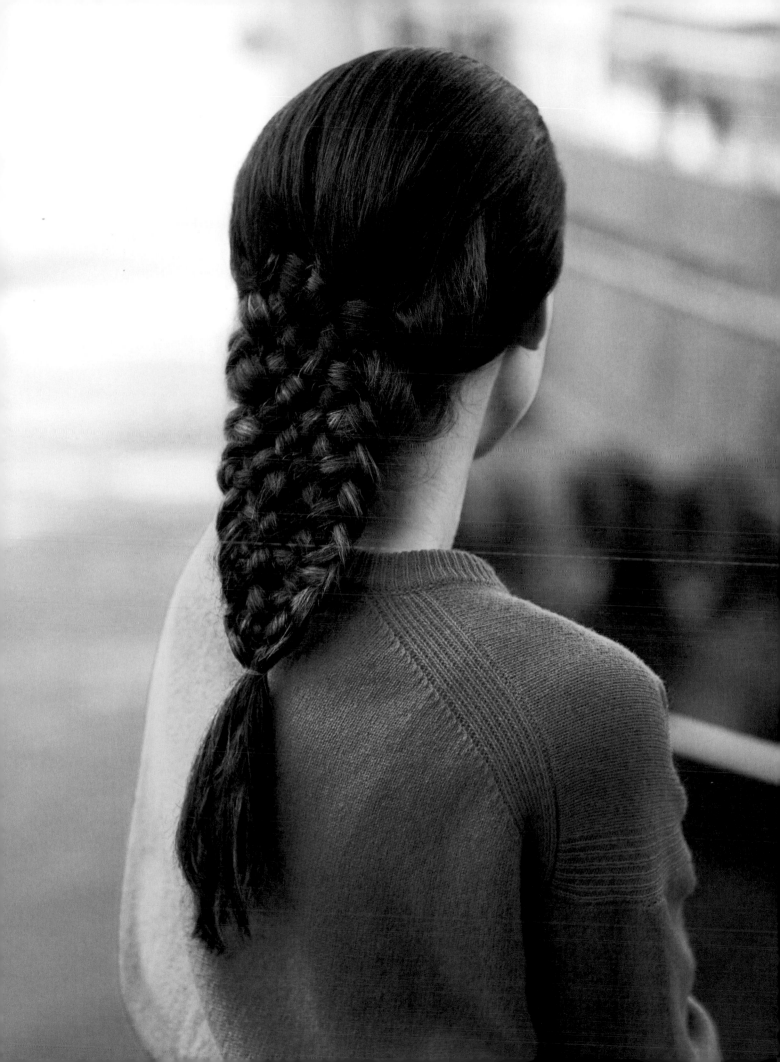

Butterfly Braid

A different and exciting braid, here a Dutch braid transitions into a feather braid. This is a hairstyle that stands out!

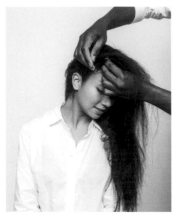

1. Brush all the hair to one side of the face. Using hairspray, brush in all wisps so that you have a smooth surface. This will make it easier when you make your Dutch braid.

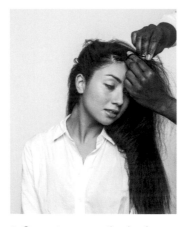

2. Separate one section by drawing a part in line with the center of the eyebrow. Divide this section into three strands. Make one round of a basic braid, crossing the side strands under the center strand. Then add in a new strand of hair with each new crossing.

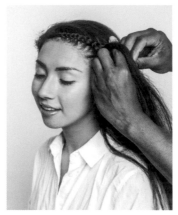

3. Alternate right and left sides by adding in new strands of hair to each section. Braid as closely to the head as possible.

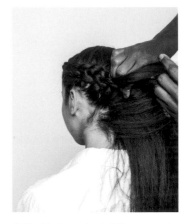

4. Braid along the hairline toward the other ear.

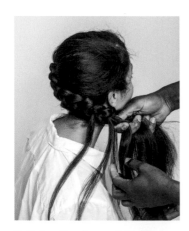

5. Follow the shape of the head. Integrate more hair as you braid. When you reach the other ear, the Dutch braid will turn into a feather braid. For each new crossing, leave out a small strand of hair that skips one round.

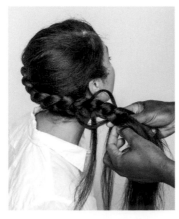

6. Add in the strands that were left hanging loose from the previous round. Now small loops will be formed as you braid. When you have finished braiding, fasten with an elastic.

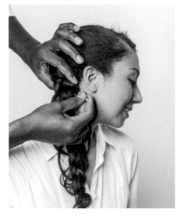

7. Insert an extra long hairpin at the side of the head to keep the braid in place. Finish with hairspray.

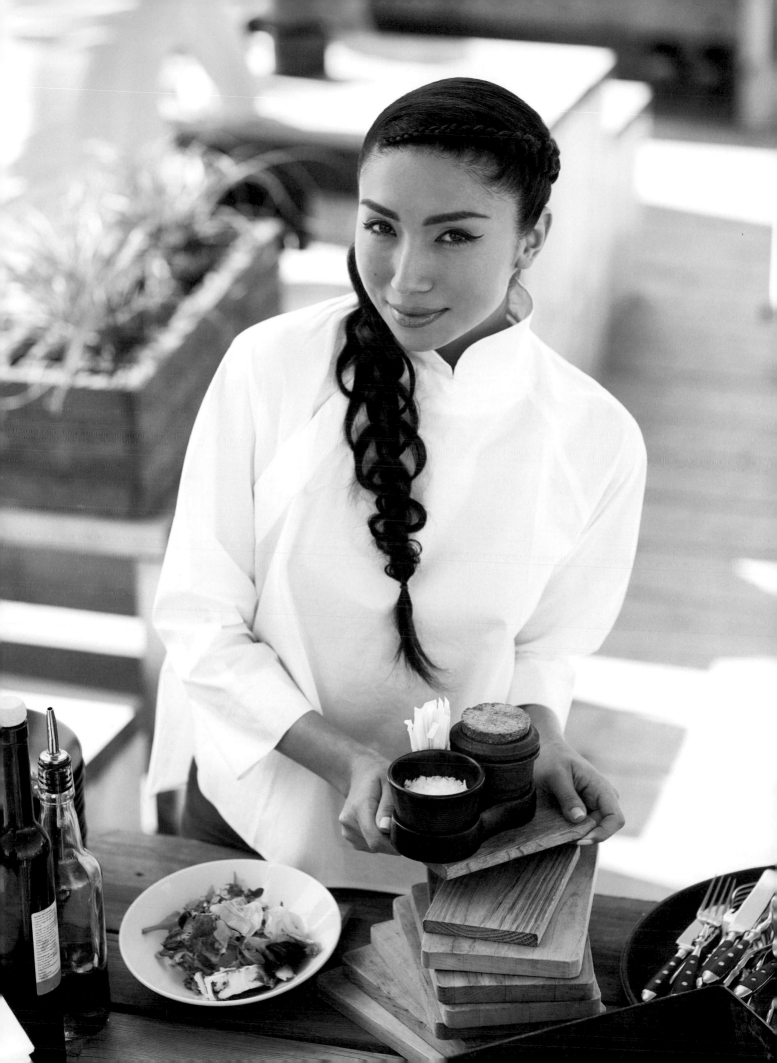

Five-Part Braid

A simple five-part braid is stylish and elegant! In this hairstyle, thin Dutch braids run down toward the neck and transition into a braid with a little extra something.

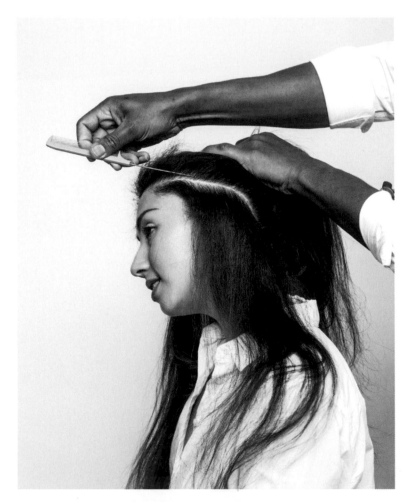

1. First, you will divide the hair into several sections. Every other section is 1.5 inches wide, and every other section half an inch wide. Begin with a 1.5-inch-wide section at the ear. Make a part from the crown diagonally down toward the neck. Keep the hair tight against the head and twist the hair toward the end. Fasten with an elastic.

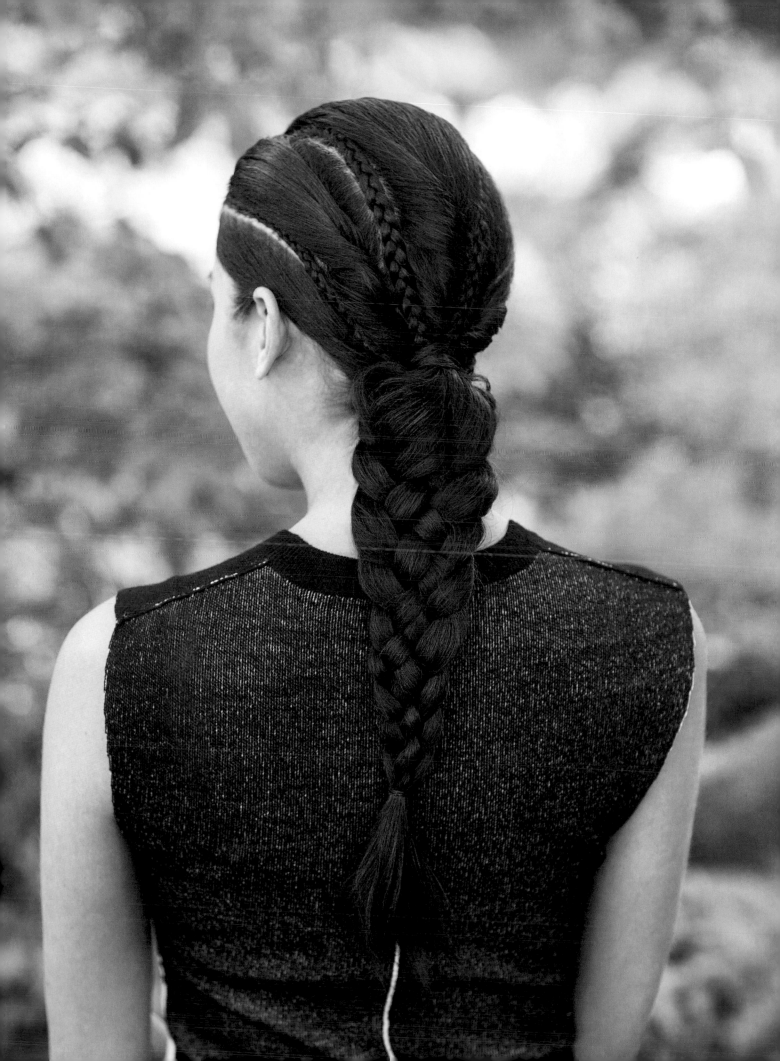

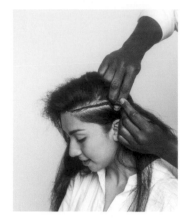

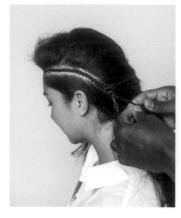

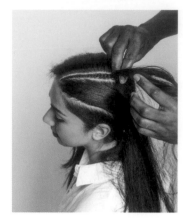

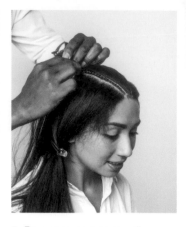

2. Draw a part from the crown diagonally to the nape of the neck. This section will be a Dutch braid half an inch wide. Divide the section into three strands. Make one round of a regular braid, where the strands are pulled under the center strand.

3. After the first round, add in a new strand of hair from the outer edges each time you make a new crossing. Alternate right and left sides by adding in new strands to each section. Repeat until the entire length is braided.

4. The next section will be 1.5 inches wide. Repeat step 1. Then make a section that is half an inch wide. Repeat steps 2 and 3.

5. Repeat steps 1 to 3 until you reach the opposite ear.

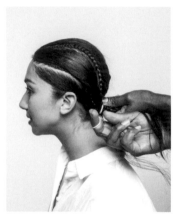

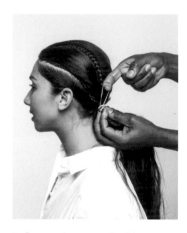

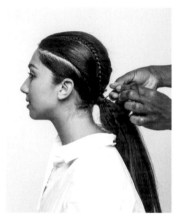

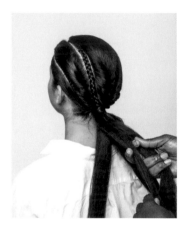

6. Gather all the hair into a ponytail. Leave out one strand that you can use to conceal the elastic.

7. Secure the ponytail with an elastic.

8. Pass the strand under the ponytail, twist it and wrap around the elastic. Secure with a hairpin.

9. Undo the braids in the ponytail. You will now make a five-part braid. Divide the ponytail into five strands.

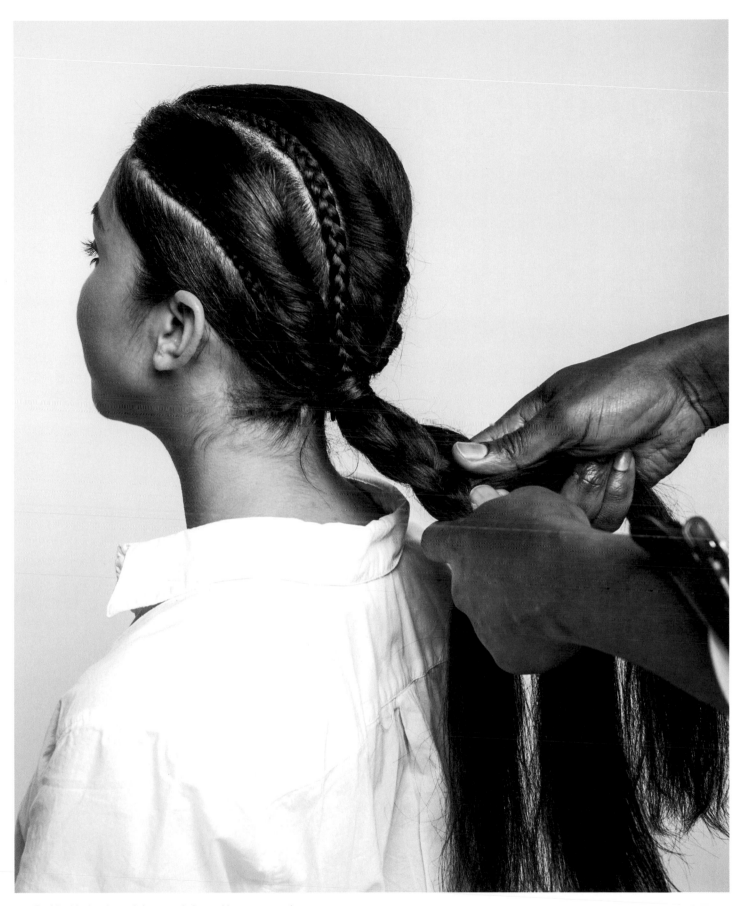

10. Braid with the three right strands by making one round of a three-part braid. Begin with the outermost right strand. Continue by braiding the three left strands, beginning with the outer left strand. Continue with the three right strands and repeat. Braid the entire ponytail. Fasten with an elastic.

Rosette Braid

Make a statement with rosette braids! This updo consists of several rosettes that run along the back of the head. The style is topped off with a high bun on top of the head.

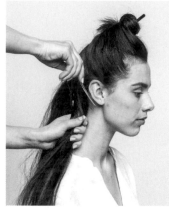

1. Draw a part from ear to ear to create a section of hair in front. Pull this section out of the way and fasten with a hair clip on top of the head.

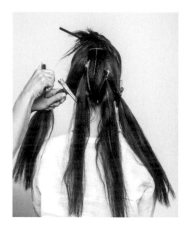

2. Divide the lower section of hair into two equal sections with a center part. Separate out two smaller sections, about half an inch wide, on each side of the center part. You now have four sections. Fasten with clips.

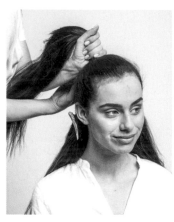

3. Gather up the front section of hair and brush it back and up, smoothing it close to the head. Use a shine cream while you work with the hair. Make a ponytail using an elastic.

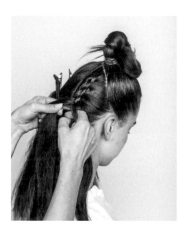

4. Begin with the right side section. Make a Dutch braid by dividing the section into three strands. Make one round of a basic braid, where the side strands are crossed under the center strand. Then add in hair from the outer edges with each new crossing.

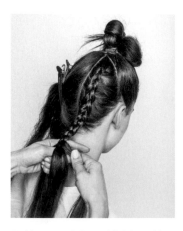

5. Alternate right and left by taking up new strands, adding to each section. After a few rounds you will see a braid that seems to lie on top of the hair.

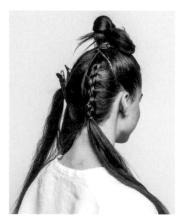

6. Braid down to the hairline and secure with an elastic.

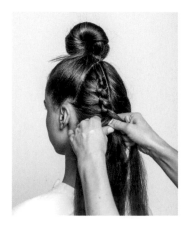

7. Repeat steps 5 and 6 for the left side section.

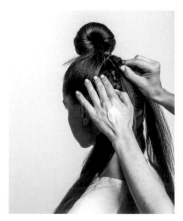

8. Using the smaller sections in the middle of the back section, you will make rosette braids. Take a strand about half an inch wide from one of the center sections. Pass a hairpin through one loop in the braid.

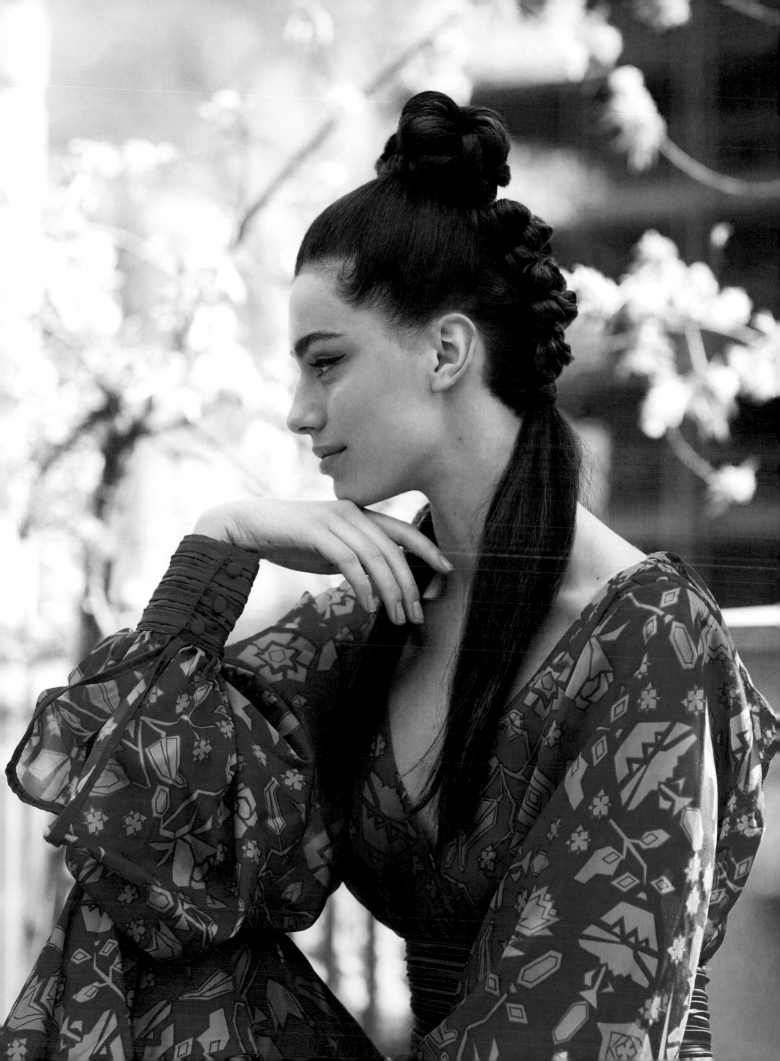

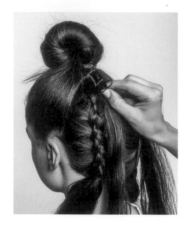

9. Twist the strand and make a loop. Pass the loop through the hairpin.

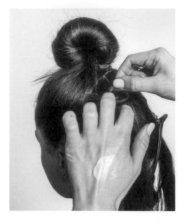

10. Pull the pin through the braid so that the hair forms a rosette.

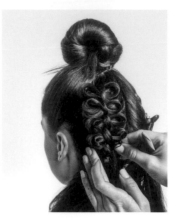

11. Repeat steps 9 and 10 as you work your way down the braid.

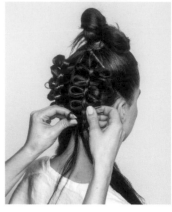

12. Repeat steps 9 and 10 also on the other braid.

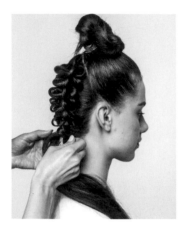

13. Twist the ends and wrap around the elastic band to conceal it, on both sides. Fasten with a small hairpin.

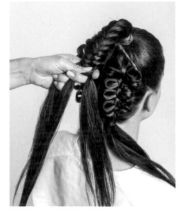

14. Loosen the high ponytail from the clip and make a fishtail braid. Divide the hair into two parts. Hold one part in each hand. Take a small strand from underneath one part. Pass the small strand around the section of hair from the outside edge and across to the opposite side. Switch sides. Always hold one section of hair in each hand. The thinner the strands that you take from each section, the more defined the fishtail pattern will be. Leave 4 inches of hair unbraided at the ends.

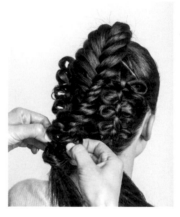

15. Pull at the braid to create volume. Begin from the bottom and work your way up.

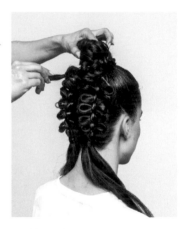

16. Wrap the braid around the base of the ponytail to form a knot.

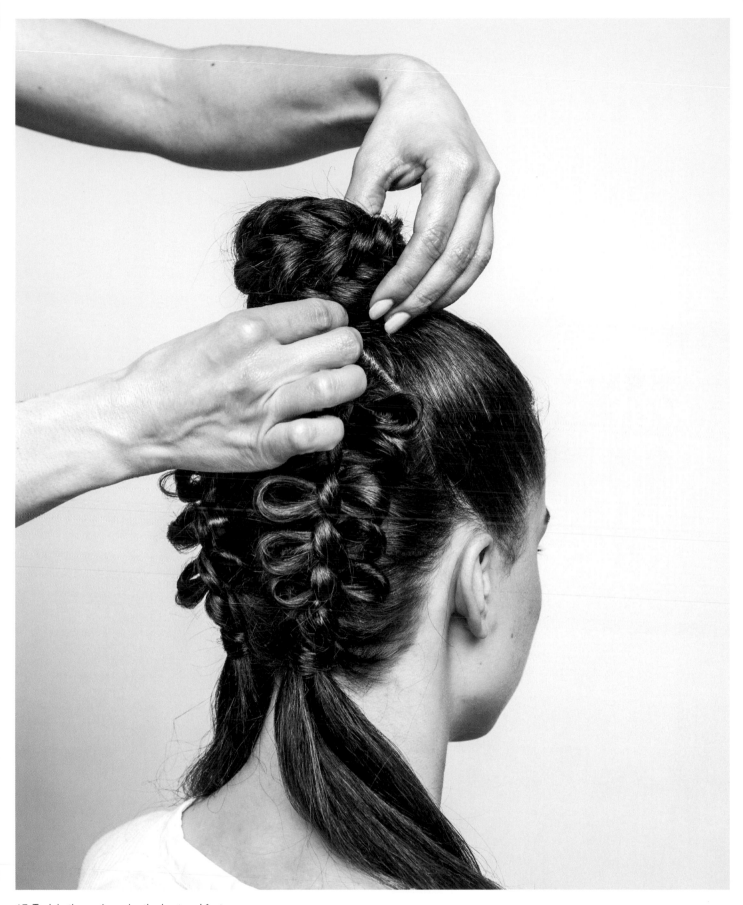

17. Tuck in the ends under the knot and fasten them with a hairpin.

Pretzel

An updo doesn't need to be straightlaced or perfect. Here we show a messy updo that combines several rope braids in a striking way.

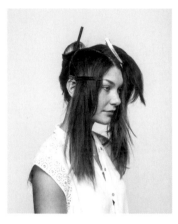

1. Divide the hair into four sections by drawing a part from ear to ear, forming a rear section. Fasten with a hairclip. Using a rattail comb, make a .75-inch-wide section on the very top of the head. Fasten the middle and side sections with hair clips.

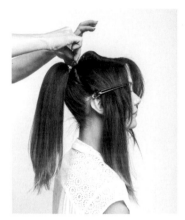

2. Gather the rear section and brush the hair upward, close to the head. Make a stable ponytail using an elastic.

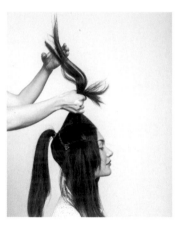

3. You will now make a French rope braid with the center section.

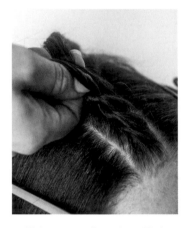

4. Pick up a small section of hair at the very front and divide it into two strands. Twist the right strand inward. Switch sides by crossing the left strand over the right. Add in hair from the remaining loose hair. Now twist the right, new hair section inward. Repeat, adding new hair for each crossing, until a rope-shaped braid is formed.

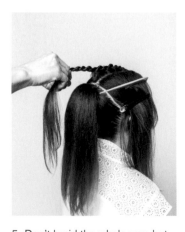

5. Don't braid the whole way, but leave the ends free.

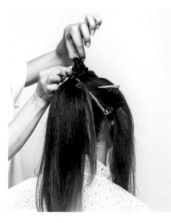

6. Pull at the lower part of the braid to create an angle.

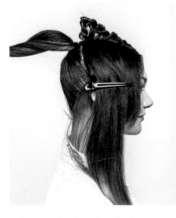

7. Fasten the braid to the base of the ponytail so that the hair forms a sharp triangle. Tuck the ends into the ponytail behind the braid.

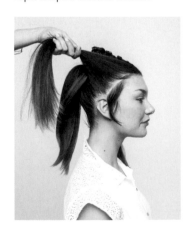

8. Gather one side section toward the ponytail, close to the head. Leave some hair free at the ear if you wish.

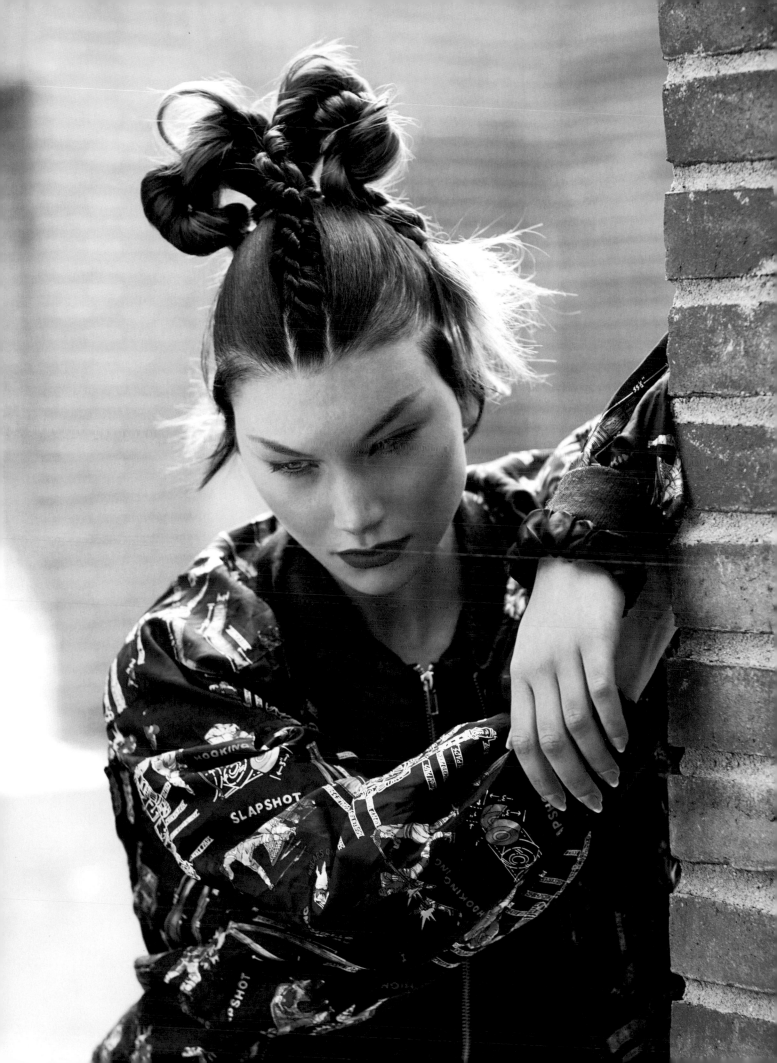

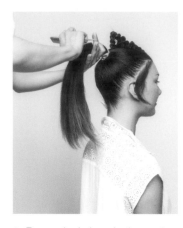

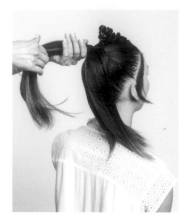

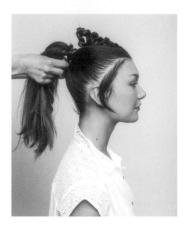

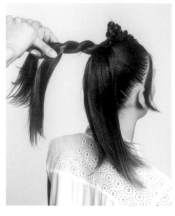

9. Fasten the hair at the base of the ponytail using an elastic.

10. Gather the other side section toward the ponytail in the same way as in step 8. Fasten hair into the ponytail in the same way as in step 9.

11. Brush through the ponytail. Take a strand and twist it. Wrap the twisted strand around the base of ponytail. Fasten with a short hairpin.

12. Divide the ponytail into two sections. Beginning with one section, divide the hair into two smaller strands. Make a rope braid. Twist the right strand inward. Switch sides and continue to twist the right strand inward. Switch places again and repeat. A rope-shaped braid will form.

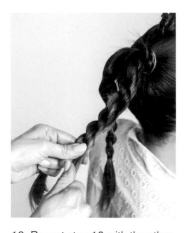

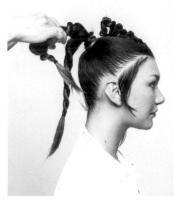

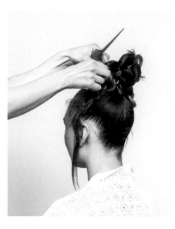

13. Repeat step 12 with the other section of hair. Fasten each rope braid with a thin elastic.

14. Fold the braids with the ends forward, toward the face. Fasten ends with hairpins.

15. Pull at the braids to create volume.

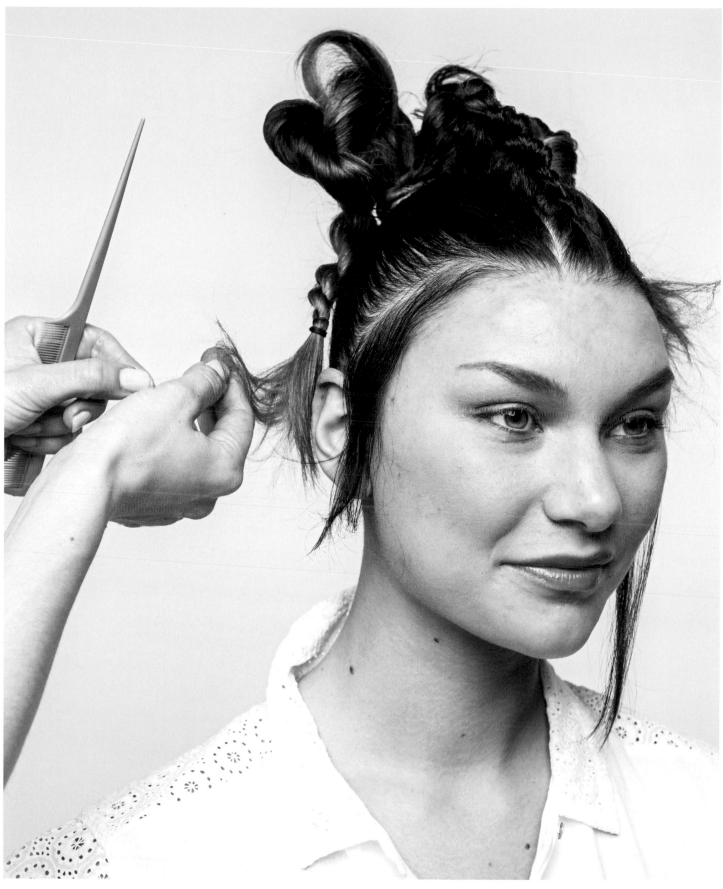

16. Tease ends with fingers. Finish with
hairspray.

Double Chain Braid

Combine a high ponytail with these stylish chain braids. This hairstyle can be worn both for everyday and special occasions!

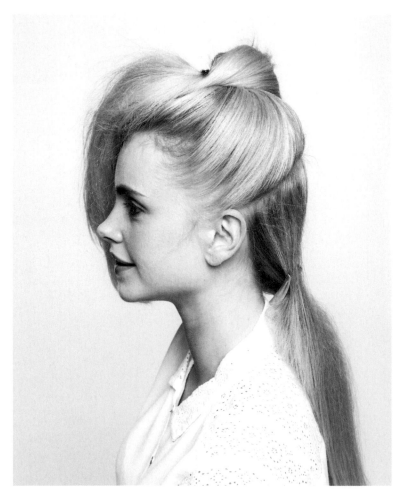

1. Divide the hair into two equal sections, an upper and a lower section.

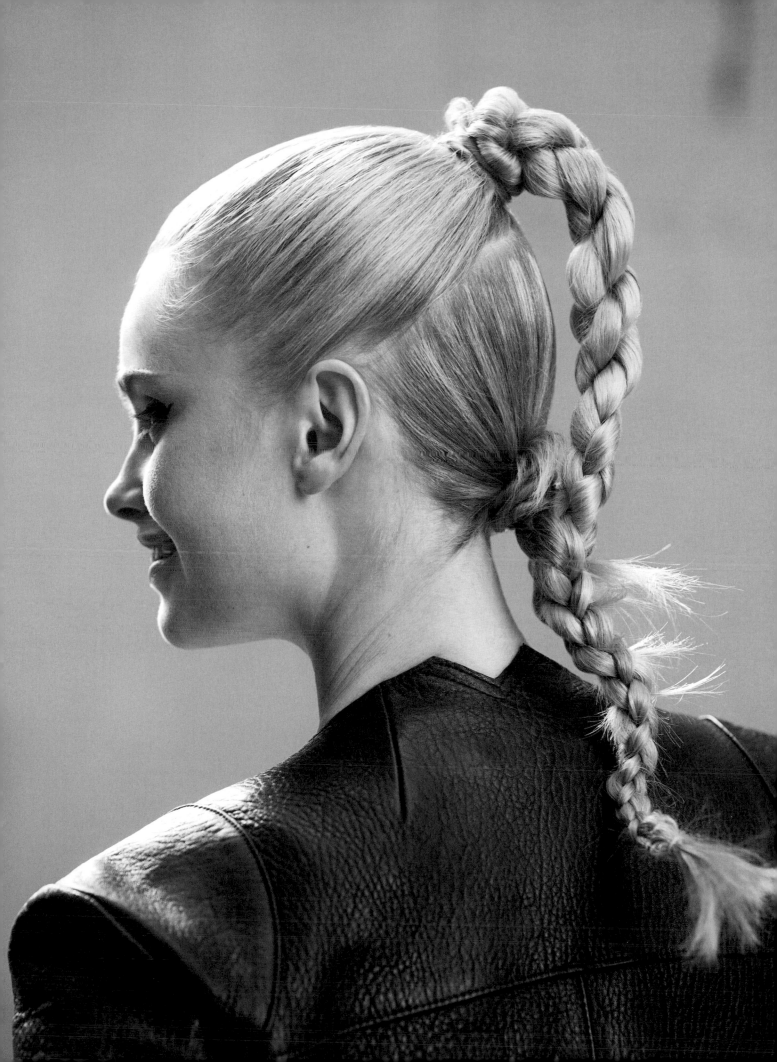

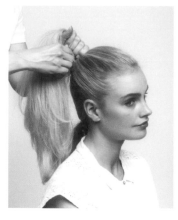

2. Gather the upper hair into a ponytail close to the head, and fasten with an elastic.

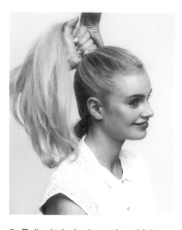

3. Pull a hairpin through a thick elastic band. Keeping the hair close to the head, push the pin right through the hair. Then wrap the elastic around the hairpin, first under and then over it until the elastic is tight. Fasten the elastic to the hairpin and then bend in the pin. This will secure the ponytail.

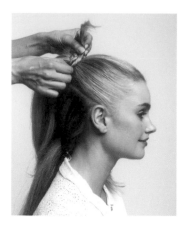

4. Take a strand of hair from the ponytail and twist it. Wrap the twisted strand around the base of the ponytail and fasten with a pin.

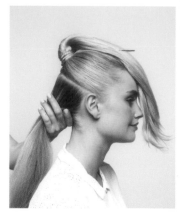

5. Now gather the lower section of hair into a ponytail, down close to the neck. Make a tight ponytail using an elastic.

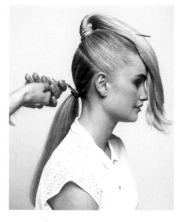

6. Take a strand of hair from the ponytail and twist it. Wrap the twisted strand around the base of the ponytail and fasten with a hairpin.

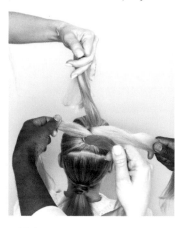

7. Make a chain braid with the upper ponytail. You will need an extra pair of hands. Divide the ponytail into two sections. Divide each into two smaller upper and lower sections. Each person holds two sections and takes turns braiding.

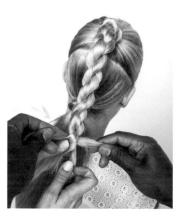

8. Cross the small sections of hair, alternating horizontal and vertical crossings. Continue to braid down toward the other ponytail.

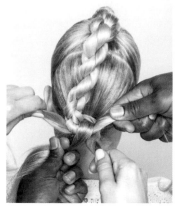

9. When the braid reaches the other ponytail, repeat step 7 and begin integrating this hair into the braid as well. Continue braiding as described in step 8.

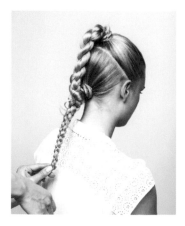

10. Fasten the braid with an elastic.

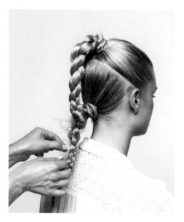

11. It's fine if some bits of hair end up outside of the braid. This adds some movement to the hairstyle. Tease lightly with fingers.

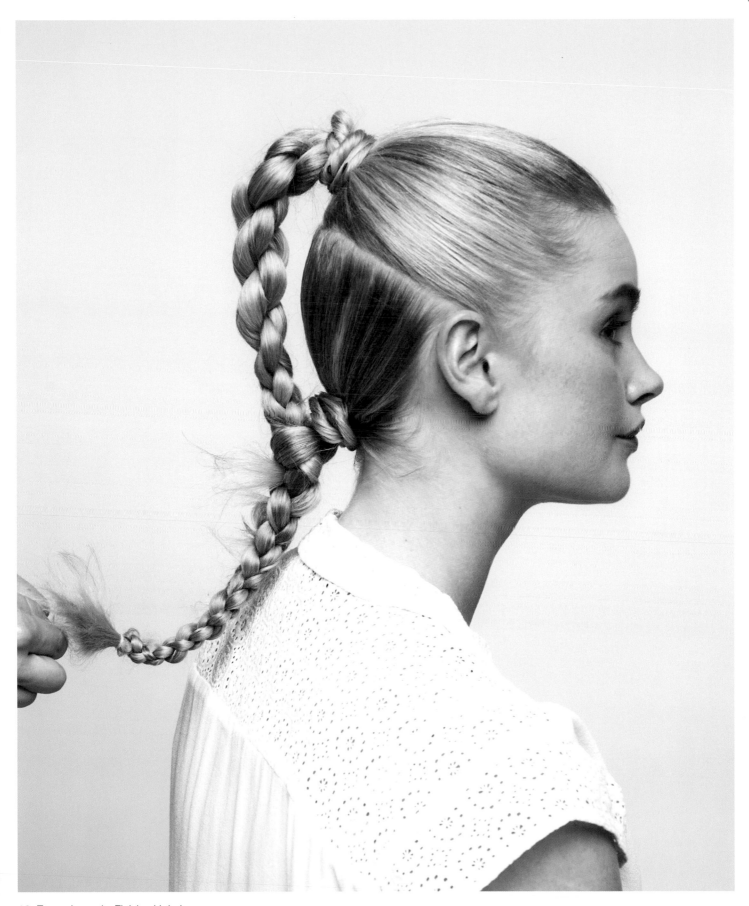

12. Tease the ends. Finish with hairspray.

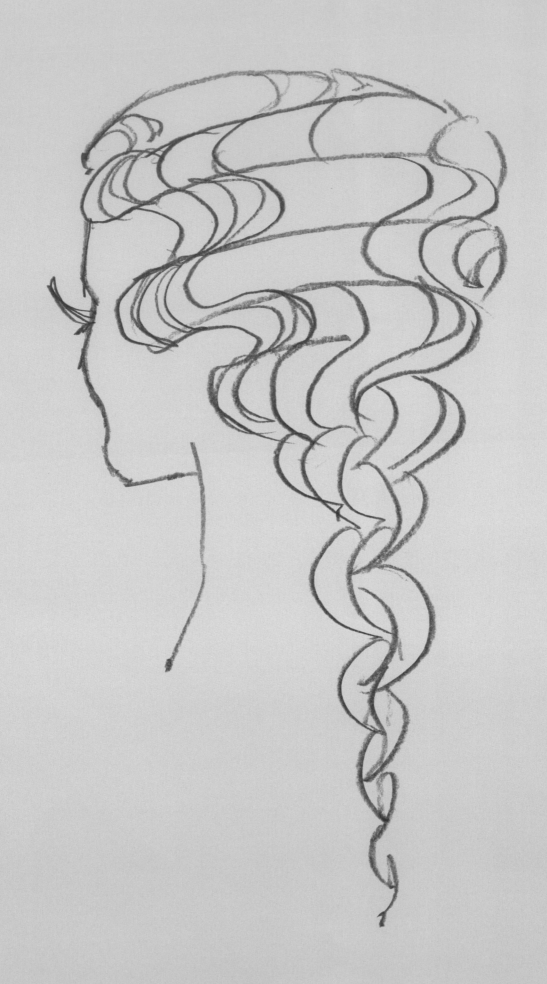

Advanced Braids

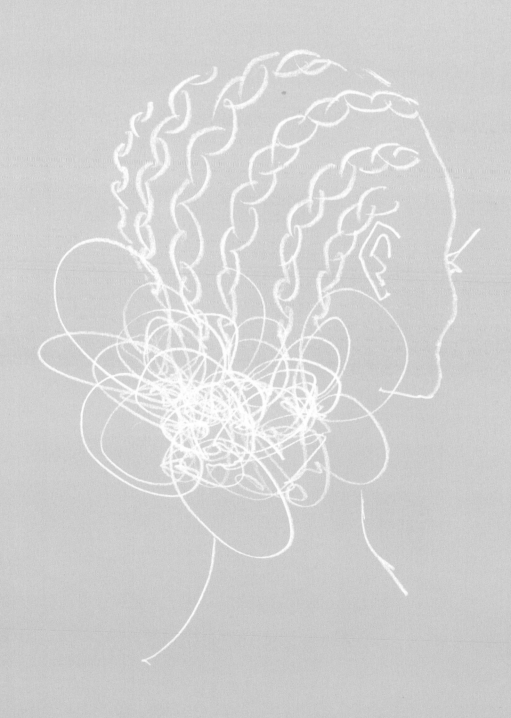

Wave Braid

The wave braid is a striking hairstyle made with many small braids that form cornrows, thereby creating a stylish and unique pattern.

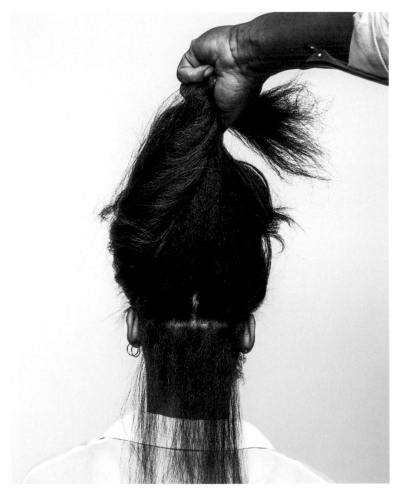

1. Separate out a section of hair at the neck and fasten with a clip.

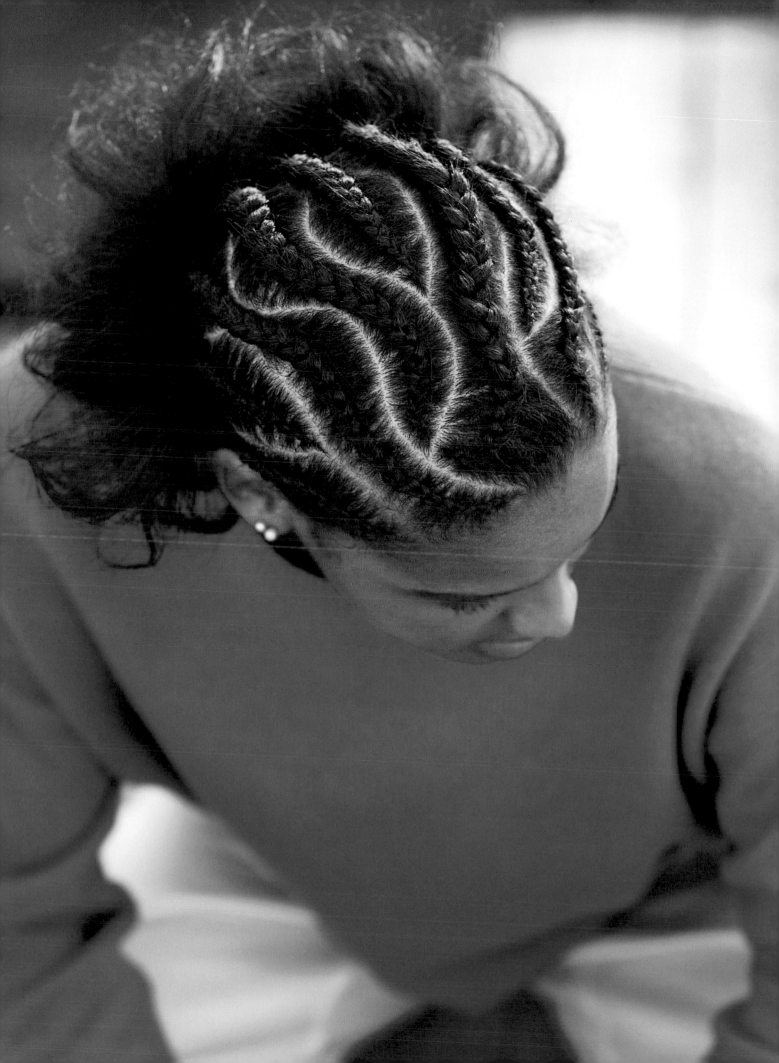

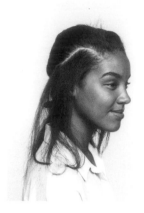

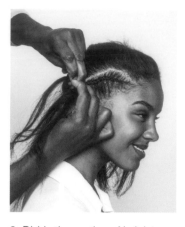

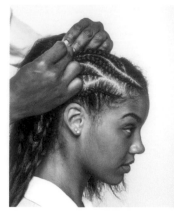

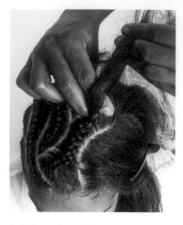

2. Brush through the rest of the hair. Using a rattail comb, make a part on one side of the head in the shape of a soft wave. The part should run from the highest point of the eyebrow down toward the neck. This style will consist of many Dutch braids.

3. Divide the section of hair into three strands. Make one round of a basic braid, where the side strands are crossed under the center strand. After the first row, add in a new strand of hair from the outer edges with each new crossing. Alternate right and left sides by adding in hair to each section. After a few rounds you will have a braid that seems to lie on top of the hair. Repeat until the entire length is braided and fasten with a thin elastic.

4. Continue braiding the hair in sections, 1 to 1.25 inches wide.

5. Wave-shaped parts create a feeling of movement and a unique pattern that can vary from one person to the next. Think of working close to the scalp so that the braid is tight and runs close to the head.

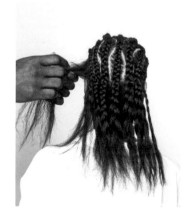

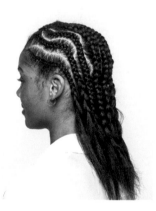

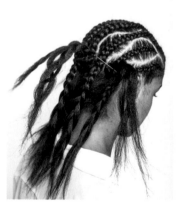

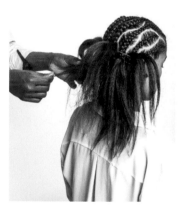

6. Repeat step 3 for each section so that the entire upper part of the hair is braided down toward the neck.

7. Stop braiding when you reach the end of the section. Fasten with a hairpin. Use a product with hold to smooth out all the wisps.

8. Create volume by lifting every other braid up a little and fastening with hairpins.

9. Undo the ends from the braid, tease, and shape the lengths with your fingers. Make sure the braids are stabilized using hairpins.

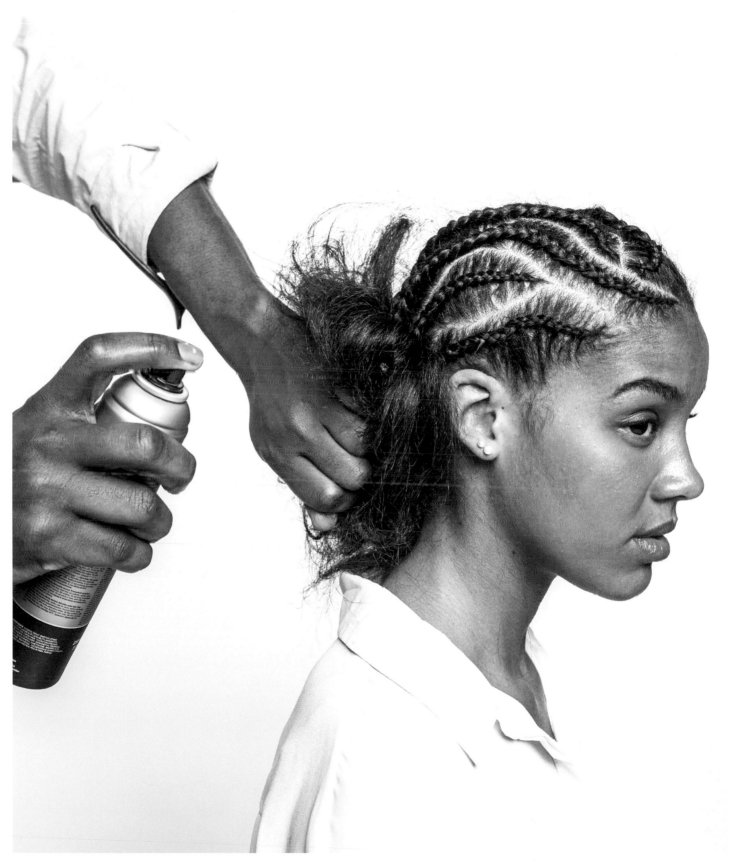

10. Play with the volume of the hair and scrunch
it upward for a messier feel. Finish with hairspray.

Rosette Bangs

Create a gorgeous look with just one braid! Here we use a rosette braid that runs like a coxcomb on top of the head.

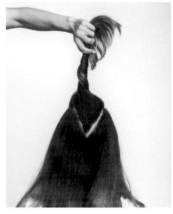

1. Divide the hair into two sections. Draw a sharp V-shaped part from the hairline down toward the neck. Section out a strand on one side of the section, about half an inch wide. Fasten the strand with a hair clip.

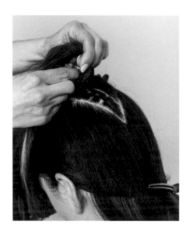

2. Using the crown hair, make a Dutch braid that runs along the head. Divide the hair into three strands. Make one round of a basic braid, where the side strands are crossed under the center strand. After the first round, add a new strand of hair with each crossing.

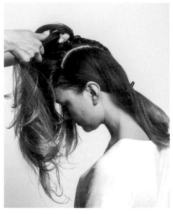

3. Alternate right and left sides by adding in new strands to each section of hair.

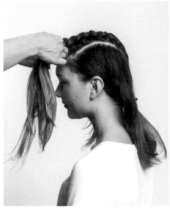

4. When you have braided all the way to the hairline, fasten with an elastic.

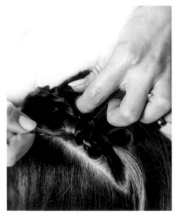

5. Pick up the strand next to the braid to make a rosette braid. Pass a hairpin through a loop in the braid. Twist the strand to form a loop and pass the loop through the pin. Pull the pin through the braid so the hair forms a rosette. Lay the ends back toward the neck.

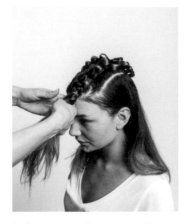

6. Repeat step 5 as you work your way forward toward the hairline. When you are finished with the rosette braid, make a few rounds of a basic braid with the ponytail.

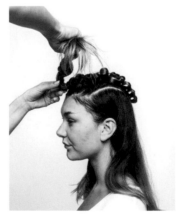

7. Wrap the ponytail around the elastic and fasten with short hairpins. Let the rest of the ponytail hang down toward the face.

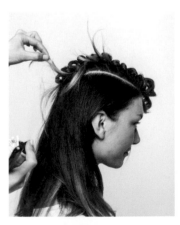

8. Pull a few strands out of the braid and let them point upward. Finish with hairspray.

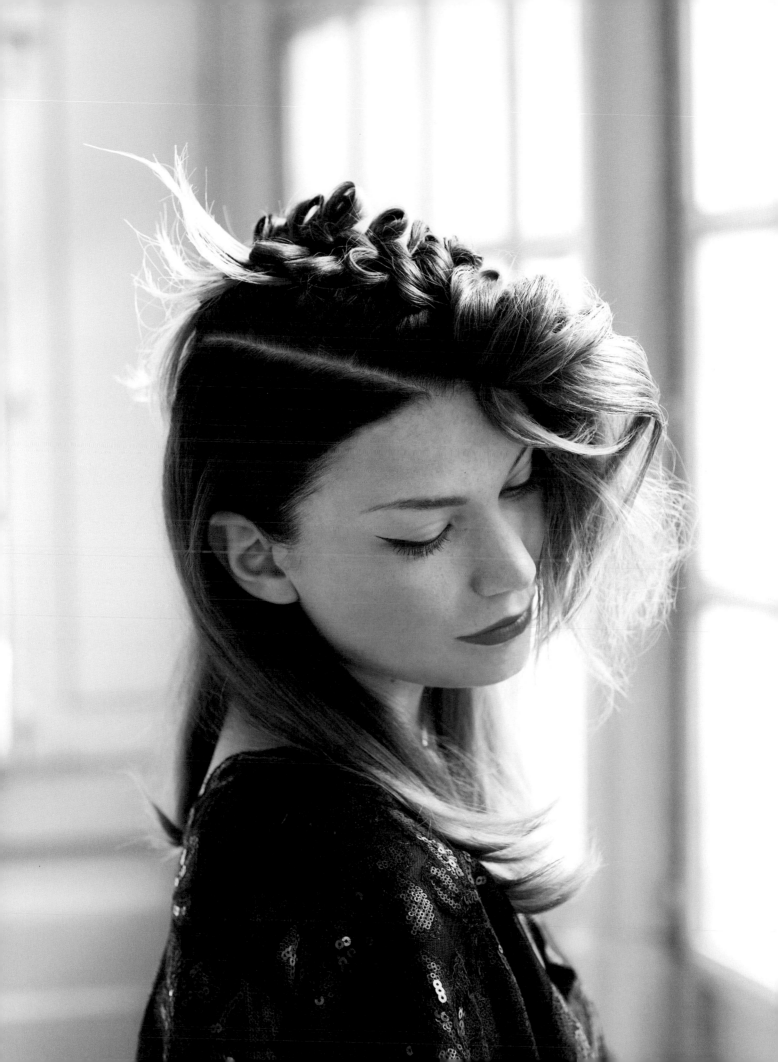

The Bow

Here we combine two four-strand braids to create an exciting shape in a hairstyle that stands out but is easy to make.

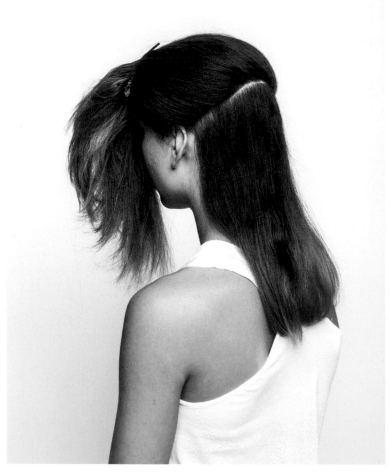

1. Draw a part from ear to ear. Pull the upper section of hair to the front and fasten with a hair clip.

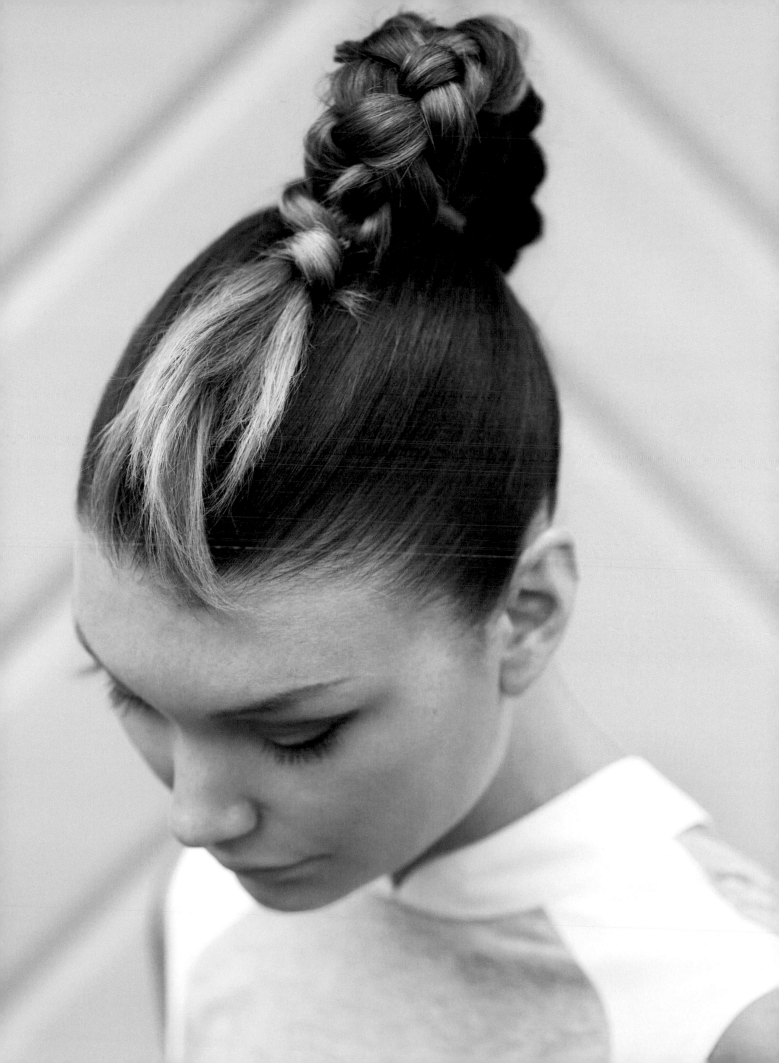

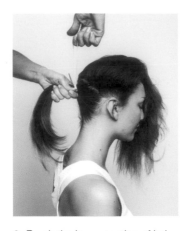

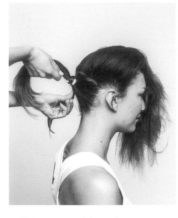

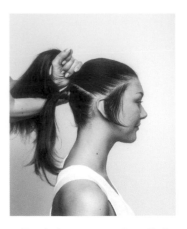

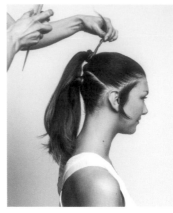

2. Brush the lower section of hair together to make a ponytail and fasten with an elastic band.

3. Take a strand from the ponytail and twist it. Wrap the strand around the base of the ponytail to conceal the elastic. Fasten with a small hairpin.

4. Brush the upper section of hair, gather it into a ponytail and fasten with an elastic.

5. Take a strand from this ponytail and twist it. Wrap the strand around the base of the ponytail in order to hide the elastic band. Fasten with a small hairpin.

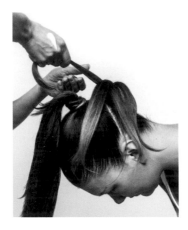

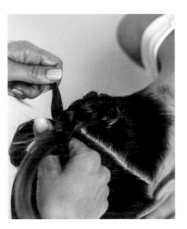

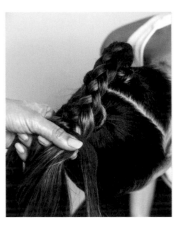

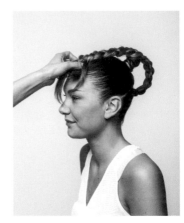

6. Bow the head down. Divide the lower ponytail into four strands. Use shine cream. You will now make a four-part braid, working upward toward the crown.

7. Begin with a regular round of a three-part braid. Begin with the three rightmost strands by crossing the outer strand over the center. Now continue by crossing the fourth strand, on the left, under and into the braid. Continue making a round of a three-strand braid with the rightmost strands by crossing the outer strand over, followed by crossing the fourth strand under and into the braid.

8. When you reach the upper ponytail, divide that into four strands as well. Integrate the strands into the rear braid and continue the four-part braid toward the hairline.

9. Leave part of the ends unbraided and fasten with an elastic.

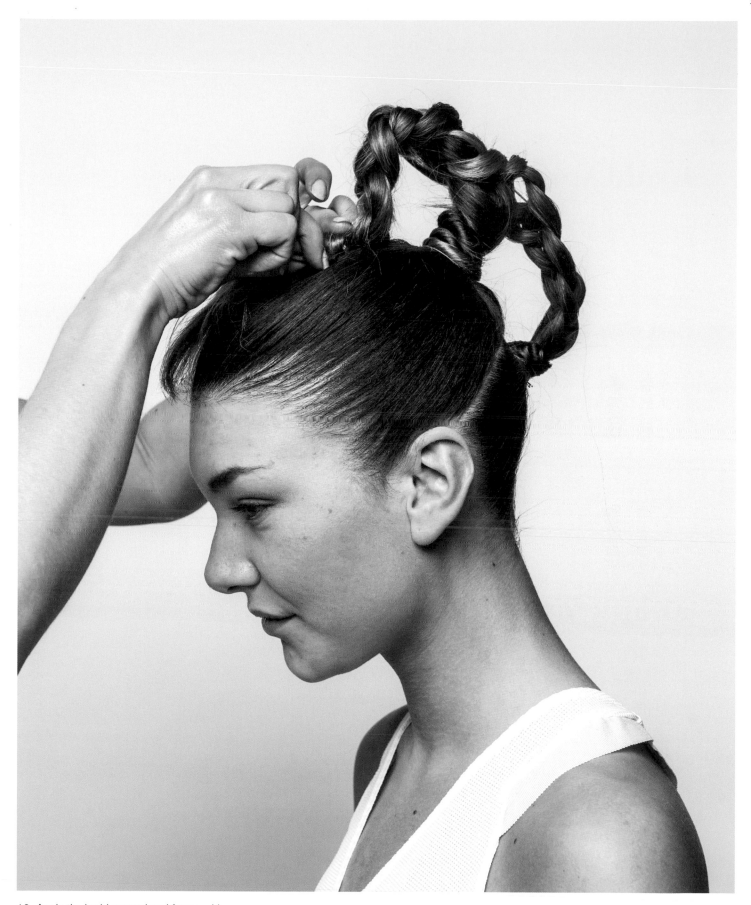

10. Angle the braid upward and fasten with
hairpins. Finish with hairspray.

Braid Models

Johanna Ågren

Freja Christianssen

Mathilda Guve

Fanny Sinyan Jernström

Moa Malmborg

Linnea Pettersson

Stina Qvarforth

Zelda Ringström

Vivi Sun

Juliet Vergara

Thank You

Thanks to Edwin Trieu, House of Dagmar, Jennifer Blom,
and One Teaspoon, for the use of their fashions.
Thanks also to these venues: Eric Ericssonhallen,
Kulturfyren, Lydmar, Restaurang Hjerta,
and the boats *Capella*, *Leo*, and *Tresor*.